Community Assessment Reference Guide for Community Health Nursing

Mary Jo Clark, PhD, RN

Hahn School of Nursing and Health Science
University of San Diego
San Diego, California

2008

PEARSON
Prentice Hall

Upper Saddle River, New Jersey 07458

Publisher: Julie Levin Alexander
Assistant to Publisher: Regina Bruno
Editor-in-Chief: Maura Connor
Executive Acquisitions Editor: Pamela Lappies
Associate Editor: Michael Giacobbe
Development Editor: Elizabeth Tinsley
Managing Editor, Development: Marilyn Meserve
Editorial Art Manager: Patrick Watson
Media Product Manager: John J. Jordan
Director of Marketing: Karen Allman
Senior Marketing Manager: Francisco del Castillo
Marketing Specialist: Michael Sirinides
Managing Editor, Production: Patrick Walsh
Production Editor: Trish Finley, GGS Book Services
Production Liaison: Anne Garcia
Media Project Manager: Stephen Hartner
Manufacturing Manager: Ilene Sanford
Manufacturing Buyer: Pat Brown
Senior Design Coordinator: Mary Siener
Printer/Binder: Courier Kendallville, Inc.
Composition: GGS Book Services
Interior Design: Janice Bielawa
Cover Design: Robert Aleman
Cover Illustration: Top, Corbis, Melanie Burford, *Dallas Morning News;* Middle, George Dodson; Bottom, Photodisk; Background, Jupiter Images, Biran Haglwara
Cover Printer: Phoenix Color

Pearson Education LTD.
Pearson Education Australia PTY, Limited
Pearson Education Singapore, Pte. Ltd
Pearson Education North Asia Ltd
Pearson Education Canada, Ltd.
Pearson Educación de Mexico, S.A. de C.V.
Pearson Education—Japan
Pearson Education Malaysia, Pte. Ltd
Pearson Education, Upper Saddle River, New Jersey

PEARSON
Prentice Hall

10 9 8 7 6 5 4 3 2 1
ISBN-13: 978-0-13-240400-6
ISBN: 0-13-240400-1

CONTENTS

INTRODUCTION

The tools included in this book are intended to assist community health nurses to provide outstanding care to individuals, families, and population groups. The tools generally reflect the dimensions of health from the dimensions model of community health nursing and are designed to be used in conjunction with *Community Health Nursing: Advocacy for Population Health*, Fifth Edition. The chapter numbers included beside each tool indicate the related chapter in the main text.

The tools may also be used independently by students or practicing community health nurses. Many of the tools are preceded by a description of the tool, the types of clients/populations for which it is appropriate, sources of data and data collection strategies for completing the tool, and potential uses of the information gleaned from the tool. Some of the tools are designed for use with individual clients or families and others for assessing population groups. Many of the tools can be adapted for use with either individuals or population groups.

Two types of tools are provided: assessment tools and inventories. Assessment tools provide guidance for assessing the health status of individual clients or population groups and provide space for recording data collected. These tools also provide direction for developing nursing diagnoses, planning interventions, and evaluating the outcomes of care. Inventories are checklists of client/population-specific interventions or risk factors for selected community health problems. Both types of tools often use the dimensions of health as the organizing framework and address relevant features of the biophysical, psychological, physical environmental, sociocultural, behavioral, and health system dimensions. Intervention guidelines in the assessment tools address the three dimensions of health care: primary prevention, secondary prevention, and tertiary prevention. In the interests of space and cost-effectiveness, duplicate pages within tools are not reproduced, but the reader is referred back to the appropriate pages in an earlier tool.

These tools provide an organizing framework to facilitate community health nursing practice with the individuals, families, and population groups most commonly encountered by community health nurses.

POLITICAL ASTUTENESS INVENTORY*

Place a check mark next to those items for which your answer is "yes." Then give yourself one point for each check mark. After completing the inventory, compare your total score with the scoring criteria at the end of the inventory.

____ 1. I am registered to vote.
____ 2. I know where my voting precinct is located.
____ 3. I voted in the last general election.
____ 4. I voted in the last two elections.
____ 5. I recognized the names of the majority of candidates on the ballot at the last election.
____ 6. I was acquainted with the majority of issues on the ballot at the last election.
____ 7. I stay abreast of current health issues.
____ 8. I belong to the state professional or student nurses' organization.
____ 9. I participate (committee member, officer, etc.) in that organization.
____ 10. I attended the most recent meeting of my district nurses' association.
____ 11. I attended the last state or national convention held by my organization.
____ 12. I am aware of at least two issues discussed and the stands taken at that convention.
____ 13. I read literature published by my state nurses' association, professional magazines, or other literature on a regular basis to stay abreast of current health issues.
____ 14. I know the names of my state senators in Washington, DC.
____ 15. I know the names of my representatives in Washington, DC.
____ 16. I know the name of the state senator from my district.
____ 17. I know the name of the representative from my district.
____ 18. I am acquainted with the voting record of at least one of the above in relation to a specific health issue.
____ 19. I am aware of the stand taken by at least one of the above on one current health issue.
____ 20. I know whom to contact for information about health-related policy issues at the state or federal level.
____ 21. I know whether my professional organization employs lobbyists at the state or federal level.
____ 22. I know how to contact that lobbyist.
____ 23. I support my state professional organization's political arm.
____ 24. I actively supported a candidate for the U.S. or state Senate or House of Representatives (Assembly) (campaign contribution, campaigning service, wore a button, or other) during the last election.
____ 25. I have written regarding a health issue to one of my state or national representatives in the last year.
____ 26. I am personally acquainted with a senator or representative or a member of his or her staff.
____ 27. I serve as a resource person for one of my representatives or his or her staff.
____ 28. I know the process by which a bill is introduced in my state legislature.
____ 29. I know which senators or representatives are supportive of nursing.
____ 30. I know which House and Senate committees usually deal with health-related issues.
____ 31. I know the committees on which my representatives hold membership.
____ 32. I know of at least two issues related to my profession that are currently under discussion at the state or national level.
____ 33. I know of at least two health-related issues that are currently under discussion at the state or national level.
____ 34. I am aware of the composition of the state board that regulates the practice of my profession.
____ 35. I know the process whereby one becomes a member of the state board that regulates my profession.
____ 36. I attend public hearings related to health issues.
____ 37. I find myself more interested in public issues now than in the past.

*Adapted with permission from P. E. Clark (1984). Political astuteness inventory. In M. J. D. Clark, *Community nursing: Health care for today and tomorrow*. Reston, VA: Reston.

____ 38. I have provided testimony at a public hearing on an issue related to health.
____ 39. I know where the local headquarters of my political party are located.
____ 40. I have written a letter to the editor or other piece for the lay press speaking out on a health-related issue.

Scoring

0–9 points	Totally politically unaware
10–19 points	Slightly aware of the implications of political activity for nursing
20–29 points	Shows a beginning political awareness
30–40 points	Politically astute and an asset to the profession

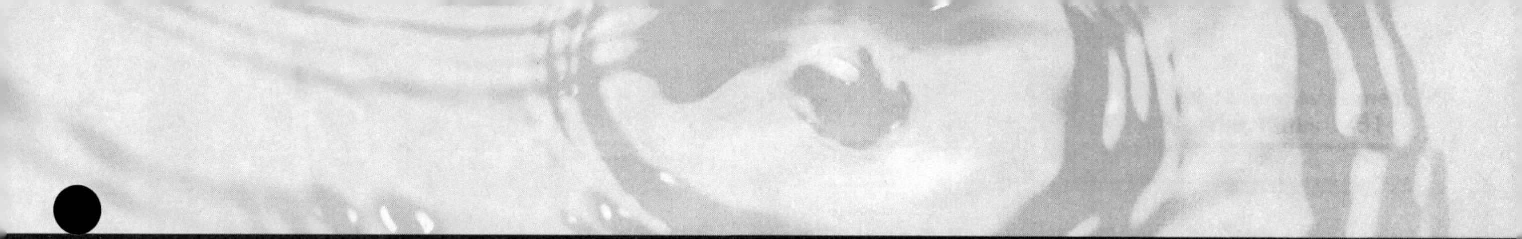

POPULATION ECONOMIC STATUS ASSESSMENT

Population size _______

Average household income _______

Percentage of households at or below poverty level _______

Composition of the low-income group:

Racial/Ethnic Group	Percentage of Poor	Age Group	Percentage of Poor
African American		Birth–1 year	
Asian		1–12 years	
Hispanic		13–20 years	
Native American		21–30 years	
White		31–50 years	
Other		51–65 years	
		66–84 years	
		Over 85 years	

Proportion of families eligible for public assistance _______

Proportion receiving assistance _______

Population unemployment rate _______

Proportion of the population with employment-based health insurance benefits _______

Annual public health funding allocation _______

Per capita personal health care expenditures _______

Percentage of people with unmet health needs due to financial constraints _______

Percentage of the population that is homeless _______

Source of payment for health care services:

Payment Source	Percent of Expenditures
Private insurance	
Medicare	
Medicaid	
Military	
Other government	
Out of pocket	
Uncompensated	

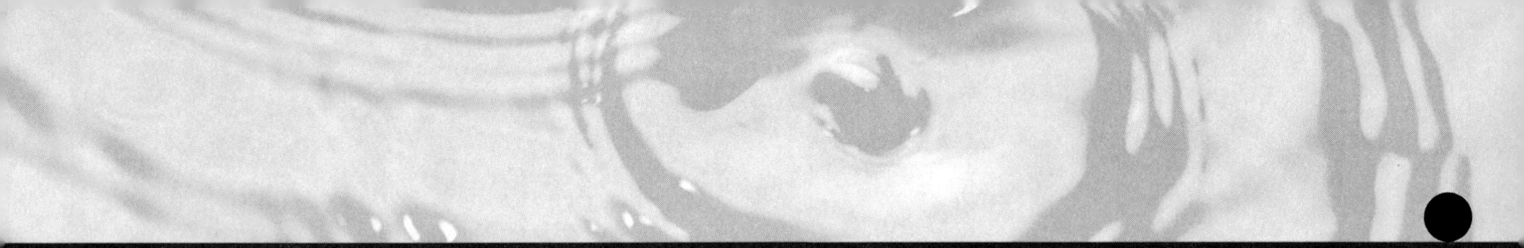

CULTURAL ASSESSMENT TOOL

Biophysical Considerations

What is the age composition of the cultural group?

Age Group	Population Size
0–1 year	
1–5 years	
6–12 years	
13–19 years	
20–29 years	
30–49 years	
50–64 years	
65–74 years	
75–84 years	
Over 85 years	

What attitudes toward age and aging are prevalent in the culture? ______________________________

____

How do attitudes toward aging affect health? ______________________________

At what age are members of the culture considered adults? ______________________________

Are there cultural rituals associated with coming of age? ______ What are the health effects of these rituals and practices, if any? ______________________________

What is the gender composition of the cultural group? ______________________________

Does gender play a role in the acceptability of health care providers? If so, how? ______________________________

____

Do members of the cultural group display genetically determined physical features or physiologic differences? If so, what are they and how do they influence health? ______________________________

____

Do group members display differences in normal physiologic values? If so, what are they? ______________________________

____

What genetically determined illnesses, if any, are prevalent in the cultural group? ______________________________

____

What are the cultural attitudes toward body parts and physiologic functions? ______________________________

____

What physical health problems are common in the cultural group? ______________________________

____

Psychological Considerations

Does the cultural group have an individualist or collectivist perspective? ______________________

How do members of the cultural group prioritize individual, family, and group welfare and goals? __________

____

What is the extent of stress experienced by members of the cultural group? ______________________

____

What are the usual sources of stress? ____

How do group members typically cope with stress? ____________________________________

____

Is there intergenerational conflict within the cultural group that contributes to stress? ______________

____

How do members of the cultural group perceive change? ________________________________

____

How do they adapt to change? ____

____

Do members of the cultural group exhibit attitudes of resignation and fatalism? If so, what effect does this have on the use of health care services? ____

____

What attitudes toward mental health and illness are held by members of the cultural group? ____________

____

Is there stigma attached to mental illness for the individual? ______ For the family? ______________

How does stigma affect health and willingness to seek health care services? ______________________

____

Physical Environmental Considerations

How do members of the cultural group perceive their relationship to the environment? ______________

____

How do members of the cultural group perceive personal space? ____________________________

What is the orientation of the cultural group to time? ________________________________

What changes in their physical environment have members of the cultural group experienced? __________

____

What influence do these changes have on the health status of the group? ______________________

____

Sociocultural Considerations

Relationships

What are the perceptions of members of the cultural group with respect to supernatural forces? ________________

____

What roles, if any, do supernatural forces have in health and illness? ______________________________

____

What are the religious affiliations of members of the cultural group? ______________________________

____

What are the major tenets of the religion(s)? ____

____

What influence does religious affiliation or spirituality have, if any, on health care beliefs and practices? _________

____

Do religious leaders have a role with respect to health and illness within the cultural group? ______ If so, what is that role? ____

Are religious beliefs and practices incorporated in health care? If so, how? _________________________

____

Do magical influences play a part in health and illness within the cultural group? ______ If so, how? __________

____

How is marriage perceived within the cultural group? ______________________________________

____

At what age does marriage usually occur? ____

Who is considered an appropriate spouse for a member of the cultural group? _________________________

____

What is the typical family structure within the culture? ______________________________________

What gender roles are expected within the cultural group? ____________________________________

____

What are the expected roles and responsibilities of couples? ___________________________________

____

How are couples expected to interact with other family members? _______________________________

What roles are typically performed by family members? ______________________________________

____

How interchangeable are these roles? ____

How congruent are family roles with those of the dominant culture? ______________________________

____

Who is responsible for decisions within the family? ____

Within the larger cultural group? ____

What are the attitudes of group members toward children? ____________________

____

What child-rearing practices are typical of the cultural group? ____________________

____

What is the typical social organization of the group? ____________________

What behaviors are expected in interactions with others within the cultural group? ____________________

____

Outside the group? ____________________

____

What behaviors are considered unacceptable by members of the cultural group? ____________________

____

What are group members' attitudes toward authority? ____________________

What is the character of interaction between the cultural group and the dominant society? ____________________

____

What is the primary language spoken by members of the culture? ____________________

What is the level of fluency with the language of the dominant culture among members of the group? ____________________

____

What other forms of communication are used by members of the cultural group (e.g., newspapers, radio, television)? ____________________

How important is context to communication? ____________________

Are there formal and informal modes of address within the cultural group? ________ In what circumstances is each used? ____________________

What courtesy titles are used and for whom? ____________________

Is a certain degree of personal reticence expected of group members? ____________________

What gestures are considered appropriate or inappropriate? ____________________

____

What do members of the cultural group expect in relationships with health care providers? ____________________

____

What do health care practitioners within the cultural group expect in their relationships with clients? ____________________

____

How congruent are expectations of relationships between members of the cultural group and scientific health care providers? ____________________

What is the quality of interaction between the larger society and members of the cultural group? ____________________

____

What is the attitude of members of the dominant culture toward the cultural group? ____________________

____

What is the attitude of members of the cultural group toward the dominant culture? ____________________

____

To what extent are members of the cultural group subjected to or perceive prejudice, discrimination, hostility, or harassment? ______________________________

Socioeconomic Status

What is the attitude of members of the cultural group toward material wealth and possessions? ______________________________

What is the educational level typical of members of the cultural group? ______________________________

What is the group's attitude toward education? ______________________________

What is the socioeconomic status typical of members of the cultural group? ______________________________

What effect does socioeconomic status have on health and access to health care services? ______________________________

Life Events

Sexuality and Reproduction

What are the attitudes of members of the cultural group toward heterosexual activity? ______________________________

Homosexual activity? ______________________________

Do group members engage in any specific sexual practices? _______ If so, what are they and how do they affect health? ______________________________

Do group members practice female genital mutilation? ______________________________

What are the attitudes of members of the cultural group toward conception and contraception? ______________________________

Is conception expected early in marriage? ______________________________

Are there special cultural practices to promote or prevent conception? _______ If so, what are they? ______________________________

Are certain behaviors expected during pregnancy? _______ If so, what are they? ______________________________

Are there behaviors or circumstances that should be avoided during pregnancy? _______ If so, what are they? ______________________________

What is the attitude of group members toward prenatal care? ______________________________

Are there special cultural practices related to labor and delivery? If so, what are they? ______________________________

Who should be present during labor and delivery? ______________________________

Where should labor and delivery occur? ______________________________

Are there special practices related to disposal of the placenta? _______ If so, what are they? ______________________________

What behaviors are expected of the mother during the postpartum period? ______________________________

What does cultural care of the newborn entail? ____________________

Who usually provides this care? ____________________

____

What are the cultural attitudes toward breast-feeding? ____________________

Health and Illness

How do members of the cultural group define health and illness? ____________________

____

Do group members hold specific theories of disease causation? ______ If so, what are they? ____________________

____

How does the cultural group classify disease? ____________________

Does the cultural group recognize any culture-bound syndromes? ______ If so, what are they? ____________________

____

What are the characteristic features of culture-bound syndromes recognized by the group? ____________________

____

What cultural health practices are used to promote health and prevent illness? ____________________

____

____

What health practices are used to restore health when illness occurs? ____________________

____

What home remedies, if any, do members of the cultural group employ to treat health problems? ____________________

____

For what problems are home remedies used? ____________________

____

How are home remedies used? ____________________

____

What over-the-counter remedies are used by the cultural group? ____________________

____

For what and how are OTC remedies used? ____________________

To what extent are these practices used by the cultural group? ____________________

What provider-prescribed medications and treatments are used by the cultural group? ____________________

____

By whom are they prescribed? ____________________

If therapies are prescribed by multiple providers, are all providers aware of this? ____________________

What are the cultural group's preferences with respect to the type of treatment modalities prescribed (e.g., massage, medications in liquid or tablet form)? ____________________

____

What measures are used by members of the cultural group to deal with the consequences of long-term health problems (e.g., pain relief, mobility limitation)? ______

Are any of the cultural practices used by group members potentially harmful? ______

Death and Dying

What are the attitudes of the cultural group toward death? ______

Do group members believe in an afterlife? ______ If so, what effect does this belief have on attitudes toward death and dying? ______

Is death a topic discussed by members of the cultural group? ______ By whom? ______

Do group members wish to be informed of life-threatening illness? ______

What is the group's attitude toward advanced directives? ______

Where should death occur? ______

Who should be present at the time of a family member's death? ______

Who should be involved in preparation of the body after death? ______

What is the typical mode of disposal of the body after death? ______

Are there special practices related to grief and mourning? ______ If so, what are they? ______

Who should participate in rituals and practices related to death? ______

Other

Have members of the cultural group experienced other significant life events (e.g., immigration)? ______

If so, was immigration voluntary or forced? ______

What are the effects of immigration or other significant events on the health of group members? ______

Behavioral Considerations

What dietary practices are typical of members of the cultural group? ______

What are the preferred foods? ______

How are foods typically prepared? ______

Are any foods proscribed within the cultural group? ______

Do certain food or dietary practices (e.g., fasting) have religious significance for members of the cultural group? ______ If so, what are they and what is their significance? ______

What is the effect of acculturation on dietary practices? ______

What are the other consumption patterns of the cultural group (e.g., tobacco, alcohol, and drug use; caffeine consumption)? ______

To what extent do members of the cultural group engage in health promotion behaviors? ______

To what extent do members of the cultural group engage in safety behaviors? ______

Health System Considerations

What alternative health systems are operant within the culture? ______

What are the characteristic aspects of alternative health systems? ______

From whom do members of the cultural group typically seek advice on health promotion and illness prevention? ______

From whom do members of the cultural group first seek assistance with health care problems? ______

For what types of health issues is assistance sought by members of the cultural group? ______

Do members of the cultural group seek assistance from different types of providers for different problems? ______ If so, whom do they seek for what kinds of problems? What is the rationale for the type of provider selected? ______

Do members of the cultural group voice a preference for providers with certain characteristics (e.g., nurse practitioners over physicians, providers of a specific gender, herbalists over biomedical providers)? ______ If so, on what beliefs and attitudes are the preferences for providers based? ______

Are there recognized alternative health practitioners in the cultural group? ______ If, so, who are they? ______

How do they learn their craft? ______

What health-promotive, diagnostic, and treatment measures do they employ? ______

To what extent do members of the group use the services of alternative health providers? ______

What is the relationship of alternative and scientific health care systems within the cultural group? ______

What is the attitude of practitioners within each system to those of the other system? ______

Are there barriers to the use of specific types of health care providers? _______ If so, what are they?___________

____

____

If members of the cultural group use multiple providers, are the providers aware of this? _______ If not, why not? ____

____

____

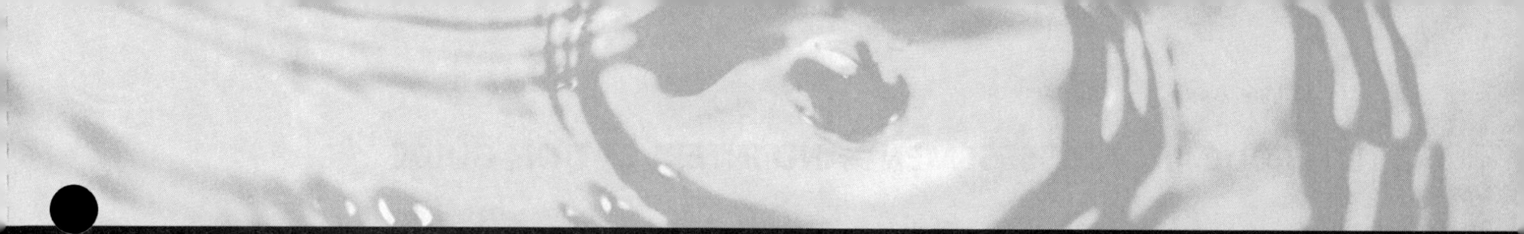

HEALTH EDUCATION ASSESSMENT AND INTERVENTION GUIDE

Description: In order to educate clients to make appropriate health-related decisions, community health nurses must identify health learning needs and then design health education encounters that address those needs. Three major elements of the learning situation should be considered: client characteristics, the material to be learned, and the setting in which learning is to take place. The tool presented here is designed to assist the community health nurse to assess clients' health education needs and to plan effective health education encounters to meet those needs.

Appropriate populations: Individual clients of all ages, groups of clients with similar learning needs.

Data sources and data collection strategies: The assessment data collected using the *Health Education Assessment and Intervention Guide* can be obtained from a number of sources. Much information about clients can be obtained in interviews with clients or significant others or from a review of existing health, school, or other records. Information regarding health learning needs may be derived from knowledge of existing physical conditions that create a need for specific learning or from learning needs typical of clients' ages. Learning needs may also be identified in interviews or client surveys or through pretesting in specific content areas. Assessment of client maturation may be derived via interviews, by observation, or from developmental testing. Information about motivation to learn and other psychological factors affecting the learning situation can be obtained from interviews, from records, and by observing clients' responses to the learning situation. Behavioral data are best obtained in interviews with clients or significant others or by actual observation of client behaviors. Information about the physical environment in which the learning encounter is to take place is most often available through direct observation. Attitudes toward health and health care or toward specific health education topics may be assessed through interviews, client surveys, or the use of attitude scales. Sociocultural information, such as education level, income, culture, religion, occupation, and so on, may be available in existing records or can be obtained directly from clients through interviews and surveys, and information about health system factors can be derived in similar ways.

Use of information: Educational assessment data allow the community health nurse to identify clients' learning needs and factors that influence the learning situation. This information then leads to delineation of specific outcome objectives for the health education encounter. Teaching strategies are selected that are appropriate to the content, to client characteristics, and to other factors that influence the learning situation. After employing these strategies in a planned educational encounter, the community health nurse evaluates learning in terms of the established outcome objectives for the encounter. Outcome evaluation may involve testing for knowledge gained, attitude assessment, or observation of learner behaviors, depending on the intended learning outcomes. The nurse also evaluates the quality of the educational assessment and the materials and strategies used.

HEALTH EDUCATION ASSESSMENT AND INTERVENTION GUIDE

Client: ______________________________ Phone: ____________________

Address: ____

Contact person (for group encounters): __________________________

Assessment of Learning Situation

Biophysical Considerations

What is the age, gender, and racial/ethnic composition of the target audience? ________________

What learning needs, if any, arise from the age and developmental level of the audience? ________________

Will the developmental level or physical maturation of the audience affect the ability to learn or the teaching strategies used? If so, how? ________________

What physical conditions in the audience give rise to health education needs (e.g., pregnancy, heart disease)? ________________

What influence will physical conditions have on the audience's ability to learn? ________________

Psychological Considerations

Is the target population aware of the need for health education? ________________

What is the level of readiness and motivation to learn among members of the target audience? ________________

Will audience attitudes toward health and health behaviors enhance or detract from learning ability? ________________

What psychological factors may impede learning (*stress, anxiety, depression, confusion, disorientation*)? ________________

What are the coping abilities of the target audience? ________________

How might coping abilities influence learning? ________________

Physical Environmental Considerations

Do physical environmental conditions give rise to health education needs? ________ If so, what are they? ________________

What is the physical environment for learning (*noise, light levels, distractions*)? ________________

Sociocultural Considerations

What effects will the learners' peers have on motivation to learn? ______

What is the education level of the target audience? ______

What prior exposure to health information have members of the target audience had? ______

______

What is the socioeconomic level of the target audience? ______

Are there cultural or religious beliefs and practices that are likely to influence learning? ______

______

What is the primary language spoken by members of the target audience? ______

What is their degree of facility with the dominant language? ______

Do the occupations of the target audience give rise to the need for health education? ______ If so, in what way?

______

______

What is the level of social support for healthy behavior in the target audience (*peer interactions, role models*)?

______

Are there other facets of the social situation (e.g., SES, time for or transportation to educational opportunities) that may influence health education? ______ If so, what effects will these factors have? ______

______

Behavioral Considerations

Do consumption patterns prevalent in the target audience give rise to a need for health education (e.g., diet, tobacco use, alcohol or drug use)? ______ What are these consumption patterns? ______

______

Do other behaviors give rise to the need for health education (e.g., safety practices, sexual behavior, need for immunizations)? ______

______

Health System Considerations

Do local health care providers emphasize health education? ______

______

Do members of the target audience have access to health care services where they might receive health education? ______

Does the target audience have a need for education regarding the use of health care services? ______

______

What is the target audience's level of knowledge of available health care resources? ______

______

Do health care recommendations give rise to a need for health education? ______

______

Are there elements of the health care regimen that may influence learning abilities (e.g., medications)? ____________

____

Will attitudes toward health care services and providers influence the ability to learn? ________ If so, how? ________

____

Planning and Implementing the Health Education Encounter

Educational Diagnoses

1.
2.
3.
4.
5.

Learning Objectives and Learning Domains Addressed

Learning Objective	Learning Domain
1.	1.
2.	2.
3.	3.
4.	4.
5.	5.

Teaching Strategies and Rationale

Teaching Strategy	Rationale
1.	1.
2.	2.
3.	3.
4.	4.
5.	5.

Plan for Outcome Evaluation

1. Measures for objective 1:
2. Measures for objective 2:
3. Measures for objective 3:
4. Measures for objective 4:
5. Measures for objective 5:

Evaluation of Health Education Encounter

Evaluation of Learning Outcomes

Objective	Status (Met/Unmet)	Evidence

Process evaluation methods and findings: ____________________

____

____

____

____

____

Revisions needed: ____________________

____

____

____

____

CLIENT DISCHARGE ASSESSMENT

Description: Case management is often initiated when clients are being discharged from a health care facility or institution with continuing care needs. The tool presented here is intended to be used to identify client discharge needs and to direct planning to meet those needs.

Appropriate populations: Clients being discharged from an acute care setting to community health nursing services, or clients being discharged from community health nursing services to other agencies or to self-care.

Data sources and data collection strategies: Data needed for effective discharge planning are available from several sources including interviews with clients, significant others, or health care personnel; health records; or observation of the client.

Use of information: Assessment data are used to identify areas in which assistance is required and to identify the care to be provided as well as appropriate sources of that care.

CLIENT DISCHARGE ASSESSMENT

Biophysical Considerations

Name: ____________________________ Age: ______ Sex: ______ Race/ethnicity: ___________________

Indicate the extent to which the client needs assistance and the type of assistance needed with each of the following functions (functional status may also be assessed using the *Functional Health Status Inventory* on pages 82–84 of this book):

Area of Function	Type of Assistance Needed	To Be Provided By
Bathing		
Dressing		
Eating		
Elimination		
Mobility		

Does the client have medical diagnoses that require follow-up?

Medical Diagnosis	Type of Follow-up Needed	To Be Provided By

Is the client on any medications? Do these medications give rise to needs for care?

Medication	Care Needed	To Be Provided By

Does the client have physical impairments that affect self-care abilities? Do these impairments give rise to the need for nursing care?

Impairment	Care Needed	To Be Provided By

Does the client have other biophysical needs that necessitate care?

Biophysical Need	Care Needed	To Be Provided By

Psychological Considerations

Does the client's emotional/mental status give rise to needs for care? ______________________

____

What stressors or stressful events are influencing the client's health? ______________________

____

Is the client able to cope effectively? ______________________

Physical Environmental Considerations

Discharge address: ______________________

Are there physical hazards in the discharge environment? _______ If so, describe them. ______________________

____

Sociocultural Considerations

Describe the client's social support network. ______________________

____

Is the client's support network adequate to meet the client's needs? ______________________

____

Are there cultural influences affecting client needs for care? If so, what are they and how do they influence care needs? ______________________

____

Does the client have needs related to the following sociocultural concerns?

Area of Need
Finances
Transportation
Social interaction
Shopping
Child care
Occupation

Behavioral Considerations

Do any of the following health-related behaviors give rise to needs for care?

Behavior
Alcohol use
Diet
Drug use
Leisure activity
Safety measures
Tobacco use
Other addictions (e.g., gambling)

Health System Considerations

What level(s) of services are needed from the health care system?

Level of Prevention	Type of Service Needed
Primary	
Secondary	
Tertiary	

RESOURCE FILE ENTRY FORM

Description: This tool is designed to assist the community health nurse to obtain pertinent data about available community resources. Many of the notations are self-explanatory, but several warrant explanation. The "resource category" notation, for example, refers to the type of agency or category of service provided (e.g., transportation, financial assistance, etc.). Funding sources may be public funds or tax dollars, private donations, fee-for-service, and so on. The contact person is a person in the agency to whom the community health nurse is known and who may be able to assist the nurse's clients with a minimum of red tape. The "source of referral" entry reflects persons or agencies from which referrals for services are accepted. For example, some agencies require that clients be referred by a primary health care provider; others accept self-referrals. The "eligibility" entry addresses criteria that clients must meet to be eligible for services. These may include residence in a particular area, certain age groups, or financial indigence. An entry should also be made regarding any fees that clients may be required to pay as well as what sources of payment are accepted (e.g., insurance, Medicaid). The "services" entry describes specific services provided by the agency, whereas "access" reflects the means by which clients gain access to the service agency; for example, whether or not an appointment is needed and how it is obtained. "Other comments" would include any other relevant information about the agency that would influence community health nursing referrals.

Appropriate populations: Community agencies (may include health-related agencies and those that only indirectly influence the health of clients, for example, employment services). Information obtained could be targeted to agencies providing certain categories of services (e.g., services to children) or to a broad range of community services that may be of use to community health nurses and their clients.

Data sources and data collection strategies: Basic information about an agency may be derived from telephone book listings (e.g., name, address, telephone number) or from existing area service directories, where available. Agency Web pages also provide a variety of information. Service directories and Websites may be out of date, so information should be confirmed in a telephone or personal contact with key agency personnel. These contacts can also elicit information that may not be included in standard service directories. Entries under "other comments" may include comments from prior clients regarding the services provided or past experiences of community health nurses in dealing with the agency. This information is best obtained in interviews with those persons who have had interactions with the service agency. Information obtained should be updated on a regular basis (at least annually or as information changes). The community health nurse may find it helpful to maintain a key contact person in each agency who will alert the nurse to changes in agency services or policies.

Use of information: Community health nurses use the information contained in the *Resource File Entry Form* to plan and implement referrals that are appropriate to a given client's situation and needs. Use of this information allows the nurse to eliminate inappropriate referrals that are frustrating for clients and service personnel.

RESOURCE FILE ENTRY FORM

Resource category: ______________________ Funding source: ______________________

Agency name: ______________________

Address: ______________________

Phone number: ______________________ Business hours: ______________________

Contact person: ______________________ Title: ______________________

Source of referral: ______________________

Eligibility: ______________________

Fee: ______________________

Services: ______________________

____

____

____

____

Access: ______________________

Other comments: ______________________

____

____

____

____

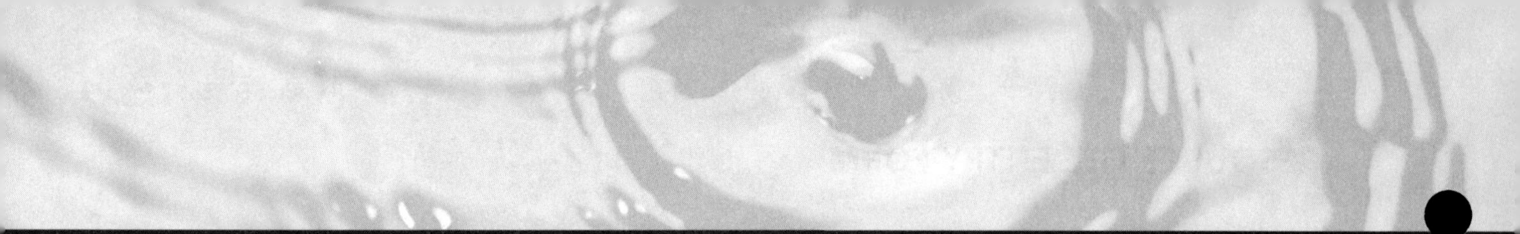

NUTRITIONAL ASSESSMENT AND INTERVENTION GUIDE

Description: Nutritional assessment involves interpretation of data from a variety of sources including anthropometric measurements, dietary history, physical examination findings, and the results of certain laboratory tests. Medication history and history of other behaviors (e.g., alcohol intake) are also relevant to nutritional assessment because of potential nutritional effects. Items contained in this tool are intended to assist the community health nurse to conduct a routine assessment of clients' nutritional status. They are framed in terms of the dimensions of health in the dimensions model. Items are *not* intended to support an in-depth nutritional assessment. In most cases, should an in-depth assessment be warranted, the community health nurse would refer the client to a nutritionist.

Appropriate populations: Individual clients of all ages.

Data sources and data collection strategies: Information can be derived from interviews with the client or significant others, medical records, anthropometric measurements, medication review, and physical examination.

Use of information: Information obtained is primarily used as a basis for health education to promote nutritional health. Information may also give rise to nursing interventions or referrals for identified nutritional deficits or other problems (e.g., obesity). Referrals may also be warranted for physical or psychosocial problems that interfere with optimal nutritional status (e.g., difficulty swallowing or depression).

NUTRITIONAL ASSESSMENT AND INTERVENTION GUIDE

Biophysical Indicators of Nutritional Status

Height _______ Weight _______ Head circumference (< age 2 only) _______

Chest circumference (< age 2 only) _______

Indicator	Yes	No	Description
Unplanned weight loss > 10 lb in 6 mo	❑	❑	
Recent weight gain	❑	❑	
Change in taste of foods	❑	❑	
Loss of appetite	❑	❑	
Increased appetite	❑	❑	
Food allergies	❑	❑	
Food intolerance	❑	❑	
Difficulty chewing	❑	❑	
Difficulty swallowing	❑	❑	
Poorly fitted dentures	❑	❑	
Sore mouth	❑	❑	
Toothache	❑	❑	
Choking	❑	❑	
Dietary restrictions	❑	❑	
Problems with food preparation ability	❑	❑	
Fatigue	❑	❑	
Fever lasting longer than 3 days	❑	❑	
Diarrhea	❑	❑	
Constipation	❑	❑	
Nausea	❑	❑	
Vomiting	❑	❑	
Dry mouth	❑	❑	
Belching	❑	❑	
Heartburn	❑	❑	
Flatulence	❑	❑	
Indigestion	❑	❑	
Increased urination	❑	❑	
Decreased urination	❑	❑	
Increased thirst	❑	❑	
Pregnancy	❑	❑	
Decubiti	❑	❑	
Recent surgery	❑	❑	
Crohn's disease or ulcerative colitis	❑	❑	
Chronic liver disease	❑	❑	
Chronic renal failure	❑	❑	
Cancer	❑	❑	
Diabetes	❑	❑	
Hypertension	❑	❑	
Cardiovascular disease	❑	❑	
Thyroid disease	❑	❑	
Anemia	❑	❑	
Hypercholesterolemia	❑	❑	
Mobility limitations	❑	❑	

Indicator	Yes	No	Description
Physical Environmental Indicators of Nutritional Status			
Inadequate facilities for food preparation	❑	❑	
Inadequate facilities for food storage	❑	❑	
Lack of access to grocery stores	❑	❑	
Psychological and Sociocultural Indicators of Nutritional Status			
Depression	❑	❑	
Mental retardation or mental illness	❑	❑	
Confusion or disorientation	❑	❑	
Alzheimer's disease	❑	❑	
Social isolation	❑	❑	
Inadequate food budget	❑	❑	
Religious food prescriptions or proscriptions	❑	❑	

Cultural food preferences: ______________________________

____

Behavioral Indicators of Nutritional Status

Fluid intake *(amount, type, frequency)*: ______________________________

Favorite foods: ______________________________

Foods disliked: ______________________________

Use of laxatives, cathartics, etc.: ______________________________

Tobacco use: ______________________________

Alcohol or other drug use *(amount, type, frequency, duration)*: ______________________________

Food preparation practices: ______________________________

Meal patterns *(frequency, timing, amount eaten)*: ______________________________

____

General food intake:

Category	Daily Servings	Serving Size	Usual Type
Grains and cereals			
Fruits			
Vegetables			
Milk and milk products			
Red meats and pork			
Poultry, fish, legumes, nuts			
Eggs			
Iron-rich foods			
Other foods (butter, sugar, etc.)			

Daily diet history:

Day of Week:

Morning meal	Time eaten:	Typical: Yes _______ No _______
Foods	Amount eaten:	
Beverage	Amount:	Typical: Yes _______ No _______
Midday meal	Time eaten:	Typical: Yes _______ No _______
Foods	Amount eaten:	
Beverage	Amount:	Typical: Yes _______ No _______
Evening meal	Time eaten:	Typical: Yes _______ No _______
Foods	Amount eaten:	
Beverage	Amount:	Typical: Yes _______ No _______
Snack	Time eaten:	Typical: Yes _______ No _______
Foods	Amount eaten:	
Beverage	Amount:	Typical: Yes _______ No _______
Snack	Time eaten:	Typical: Yes _______ No _______
Foods	Amount eaten:	
Beverage	Amount:	Typical: Yes _______ No _______
Snack	Time eaten:	Typical: Yes _______ No _______
Foods	Amount eaten:	
Beverage	Amount:	Typical: Yes _______ No _______

Medication Use*	Yes	No
Antacids	❑	❑
Antibiotics	❑	❑
Anticoagulants	❑	❑
Anticonvulsants	❑	❑
Antidepressants	❑	❑
Antihypertensives	❑	❑
Antineoplastics	❑	❑
Antituberculins	❑	❑
Aspirin	❑	❑
Cathartics	❑	❑
Diuretics	❑	❑
Hypocholesterolemics	❑	❑
Oral contraceptive agents	❑	❑
Sedatives/hypnotics	❑	❑
Steroids	❑	❑

Health System Indicators of Nutritional Status

Therapeutic diet prescribed: ______________________________

Radiation therapy: ______________________________

Chemotherapy: ______________________________

Nutrition-Related Health Problems Identified

1. ______________________________
2. ______________________________
3. ______________________________
4. ______________________________
5. ______________________________

Nursing Interventions for Nutrition-Related Problems

1. ______________________________
2. ______________________________
3. ______________________________
4. ______________________________
5. ______________________________

*Not all drugs in these categories have nutritional effects, and nutritional effects may vary among drugs in the same category. The community health nurse should familiarize him- or herself with the particular effects of specific drugs in each category.

Expected Outcomes of Nursing Interventions

1. ______________________________
2. ______________________________
3. ______________________________
4. ______________________________
5. ______________________________

Evaluation of Intervention Outcomes

1. ______________________________
2. ______________________________
3. ______________________________
4. ______________________________
5. ______________________________

FAMILY HEALTH ASSESSMENT AND INTERVENTION GUIDE

Description: This tool incorporates the dimensions model to assess the health needs of families as the recipients of care by community health nurses and to plan, implement, and evaluate that care. The assessment portion of the tool addresses factors in each of the six dimensions of health that may influence the health of the family.

Appropriate populations: Appropriate to all types of families (e.g., nuclear or extended families, blended families). May also be used with families from a variety of cultural groups.

Data sources and data collection strategies: The primary source of data will be interviews with family members and observations made by the community health nurse. The nurse may also obtain information from other persons to whom the family is well known. The nurse should, however, be sure to obtain the consent of the family before seeking information from outside sources such as health care providers, teachers, and so on.

Use of information: Information obtained in the family assessment is used to make nursing diagnoses related to family health status and to identify problems that require nursing intervention. Family problems for which intervention may be required may be more or less directly related to health. For example, a referral for financial assistance is much less directly related to health status than is providing services such as immunizations. Based on the nursing diagnoses derived from assessment data, the community health nurse plans, implements, and evaluates interventions specifically designed to fit the family's circumstances, taking into account their strengths and ameliorating areas of difficulty.

FAMILY HEALTH ASSESSMENT AND INTERVENTION GUIDE

Family surname(s): ______________________ Phone: __________

Address: ______________________________________

Assessment

Biophysical Considerations

Family composition:

Name	Age	Sex	Physical Health Status
1.			
2.			
3.			
4.			
5.			

Maturation and Aging

Are individual family members' developmental tasks met? ______________________

____

Extent of support for development of individual family members: ______________________

____

Effects of individual development on family health: ______________________

What is the stage of family development? ______________________

How well has the family achieved relevant developmental tasks? ______________________

____

Physiologic Function

Family members' current health problems and treatment regimen (*type, effects, source*): __________

____

____

Significant past health problems of family members: ______________________

____

Significant family history of hereditary conditions: ______________________

____

Immunization status of family members: ______________________

____

Psychological Considerations

Family strengths and weaknesses: ____________________

____

Family communication (*typical patterns, effectiveness, purposes, tone, rules*): ____________________

____

Extent of emotional support for family members: ____________________

____

Coping strategies used by family members (*type, effectiveness, response to crisis*): ____________________

____

Level of family cohesion: ____________________

____

Family decision mechanisms: ____________________

____

Quality of family member interactions: ____________________

____

Discipline (*type, source, consistency, appropriateness*): ____________________

____

History of mental illness in family members: ____________________

____

Family goals (*congruence with individual and societal goals*): ____________________

____

Sources of stress for family members: ____________________

____

Evidence of violence in the family: ____________________

____

Physical Environmental Considerations

Family home (*location, adequacy for family size*): ____________________

____

Safety hazards present in home: ____________________

____

Neighborhood (*safety, services and facilities available, pollutants*): ____________________

____

Access to goods and services in the community: ____________________

Family emergency plan: ____________________

Sociocultural Considerations

Family roles:

Role	Performed By	Adequacy	Role Model
Leader			
Child care			
Sexual			
Breadwinner			
Confidant			
Disciplinarian			
Homemaker			
Repairperson			
Financial manager			

Presence of role conflict or role overload: ______________________________

____

Adequacy of role performance: ______________________________

Anticipated changes in family roles: ______________________________

Role congruence with dominant culture: ______________________________

Religious affiliations of family members and their influence on health: ______________________________

____

Family cultural affiliations and influences on health: ______________________________

____

Family income (*source, adequacy, effectiveness of management*): ______________________________

____

Educational level of family members: ______________________________

____

External resources available to family: ______________________________

____

Occupation

Family Member	Occupation	Employer

Occupational health hazards for family members: ______________________________

____

Family immigration status and effects: ______________________________

Behavioral Considerations

Consumption Patterns

Family dietary patterns (*amount, food preferences, preparation, adequacy, special needs*): ______

Use of other substances (*tobacco, alcohol, other drugs*): ______

Use of prescription and nonprescription medications: ______

Rest and exercise patterns: ______

Leisure Activity

Typical leisure activities of family members: ______

Health hazards posed by family leisure pursuits: ______

Use of recreational activities to enhance family cohesion: ______

Other Behaviors

Use of safety devices and practices: ______

Safety education for family members: ______

Family planning (*need for, type, effectiveness*): ______

Sexual activity (*by whom, attitudes toward sexual activity*): ______

Health System Considerations

Family definitions of and attitudes toward health: ______

Family response to illness: ______

Health-related decision making: ______

Use of folk remedies and self-care practices: ______

Usual source of health care: ______

Means of financing health care: ____________________

Use of primary, secondary, and tertiary health care services: ____________________

Barriers to obtaining health care: ____________________

Diagnosis

Biophysical Diagnoses

Positive Nursing Diagnoses	Negative Nursing Diagnoses

Psychological Diagnoses

Positive Nursing Diagnoses	Negative Nursing Diagnoses

Physical Environmental Diagnoses

Positive Nursing Diagnoses	Negative Nursing Diagnoses

Sociocultural Diagnoses

Positive Nursing Diagnoses	Negative Nursing Diagnoses

Behavioral Diagnoses

Positive Nursing Diagnoses	Negative Nursing Diagnoses

Health System Diagnoses

Positive Nursing Diagnoses	Negative Nursing Diagnoses

Planning

Planned Interventions	Outcome Objectives

Implementation

Intervention	Responsible Party/Expected Completion Date	Status

Evaluation

Expected Outcome	Status (Met/Unmet)	Supporting Evidence

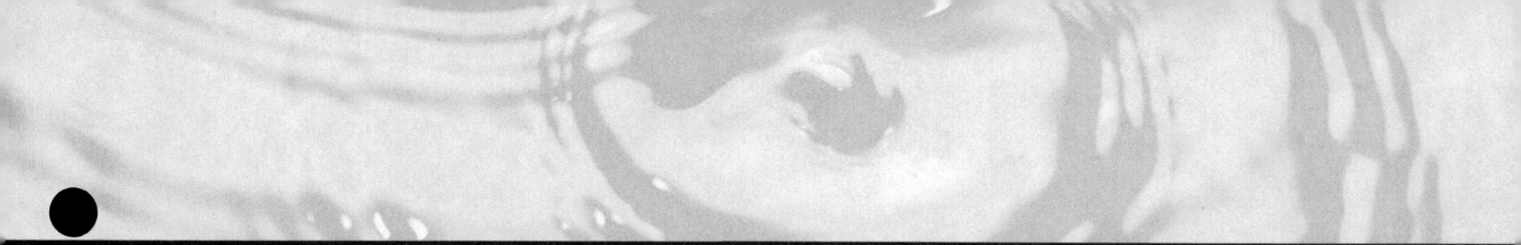

FAMILY CRISIS RISK INVENTORY

	Yes	No
Biophysical Considerations		
Are family members entering transitional periods in personal development (e.g., adolescence)?	❑	❑
Is the family entering a transition period in its development (e.g., birth of a child)?	❑	❑
Does the health status of one or more family members increase the risk of crisis?	❑	❑
Will existing health problems impede the family's ability to deal effectively with a crisis?	❑	❑
Psychological Considerations		
Does the family have effective coping skills?	❑	❑
Is the family capable of working together to resolve a crisis?	❑	❑
Do family members exhibit closeness?	❑	❑
Do family members exhibit insight into the potential for crisis in their situation?	❑	❑
Do family members exhibit insight into factors affecting a crisis situation?	❑	❑
Is the family "crisis-prone"?	❑	❑
Does the family have a history of successfully resolving past crises?	❑	❑
Does mental or emotional illness in the family increase the risk of crisis?	❑	❑
Has mental or emotional illness in a family member precipitated a crisis?	❑	❑
Are any family members seriously depressed?	❑	❑
Is there a risk for suicide for any family member?	❑	❑
Is there a risk for homicide in the family?	❑	❑
Physical Environmental Considerations		
Do family living conditions increase the risk of crisis?	❑	❑
Sociocultural Considerations		
Does the family have a strong social support network?	❑	❑
Do family interactions give rise to the potential for crisis?	❑	❑
Does the family's financial situation contribute to the risk of crisis?	❑	❑
Does the family's financial situation impede its ability to respond effectively to crises?	❑	❑
Does stress in the occupational setting give rise to the potential for family crisis?	❑	❑
Does the family have access to emotional, financial, or material support from others?	❑	❑
Behavioral Considerations		
Do any family members abuse psychoactive substances (alcohol, drugs)?	❑	❑
Has substance abuse precipitated a family crisis?	❑	❑
Does substance abuse impede the family's ability to respond effectively to crises?	❑	❑
Do family members have access to recreational and leisure activities to decrease stress?	❑	❑
Do family members engage in recreational and leisure activities that promote cohesion?	❑	❑
Health System Considerations		
Does the family have health insurance coverage to deal with a health care crisis?	❑	❑
Is the family knowledgeable about resources for dealing with factors such as substance abuse or life-threatening illness that may precipitate crises?	❑	❑
Have extensive medical bills precipitated a family crisis?	❑	❑

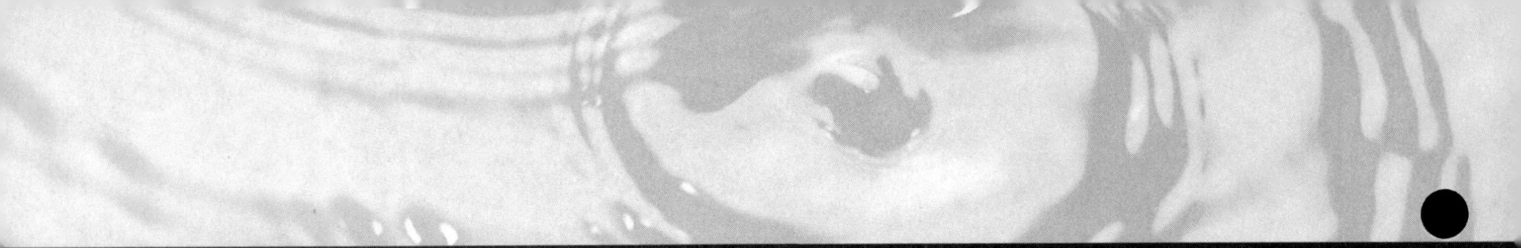

NEIGHBORHOOD/COMMUNITY SAFETY INVENTORY

Description: This tool can be used to assess physical and psychosocial safety hazards in a given client's neighborhood or in a community at large. The tool assesses elements of the physical environmental, psychological, and social dimensions of health in the dimensions model. The inventory promotes identification of safety problems in the neighborhood or community and planning of nursing interventions to resolve identified problems.

Appropriate populations: Any neighborhood or community. May also be used to assess the neighborhood in which a specific individual client or family lives.

Data sources and data collection strategies: Personal observation of the neighborhood and interviews with residents and key informants are excellent means of obtaining information about neighborhood or community safety. Examples of key informants include local police and fire personnel, business and industry leaders, community officials, local disaster planning groups, department of transportation officials, and insurance company representatives. Review of police, fire, and insurance records may also be a source of important environmental safety information.

Use of information: Information derived using the tool can be used to educate individual clients regarding elimination or avoidance of safety hazards. Information may also be helpful in planning community safety education programs, in initiating disaster planning efforts, or to support political activity to enhance neighborhood or community safety. Finally, neighborhood safety information may assist the nurse to take precautions to promote his or her own safety while working in the area. Using information derived from the inventory, the community health nurse develops nursing diagnoses related to safety problems and plans interventions for those problems. Frequently, the interventions needed will require collaboration with other agencies and individuals, but may be initiated by the nurse.

NEIGHBORHOOD/COMMUNITY SAFETY INVENTORY

Neighborhood or community assessed: ______

Safety Hazards in the Natural Environment

What is the extent of air pollution? What pollutants are involved? ______

______

What is the extent of water pollution? What pollutants are involved? ______

______

What is the extent of natural radiation in the area? ______

______

Are there other environmental pollutants in the area? ______

______

Do local weather conditions pose health hazards? ______

Are there drowning hazards (e.g., lakes, rivers) in the area? ______

Do wild animals in the area serve as reservoirs for disease? ______

Do stray animals pose a safety or health hazard in the neighborhood? ______

What poisonous plants or plant allergens grow in the area? ______

______

Safety Hazards in the Built Environment

Do residential units pose safety hazards? ______

______

What is the extent of disrepair in housing units? ______

Are there structural defects in area buildings, roads, and so on that pose safety hazards? ______

______

Do local building codes effectively address safety issues? ______

Are building safety codes enforced? ______

Are there broken sidewalks (or lack of sidewalks) or other external safety hazards in the neighborhood that pose health risks? ______

Is there a lead exposure hazard in the area? ______

How adequate is sanitation and waste disposal? ______

Is there a problem with trash or garbage that poses a health risk? ______

What is the prevalence of residential fires? ______

What proportion of homes in the area have functional smoke alarms or sprinkler systems? ______

What are the local fire insurance rates? ______

To what extent do residents (home owners and renters) carry fire insurance? ______

What is the response time for fire personnel? ______

Are area swimming pools adequately fenced? ______

What is the prevalence of traffic accidents? ______

Do traffic accidents tend to occur in specific areas? ______ If so, where and why? ______

______

What are the local car insurance rates? ______

To what extent do residents carry automobile insurance? ______

What is the response time for emergency personnel? ______

Are there significant noise hazards in the area? ______

What safety hazards are posed by local industry? ______

______

To what extent do local industries adhere to safety standards? ______

______

Safety Hazards in the Psychological Environment

How secure do area residents feel? ______

To what extent do environmental conditions contribute to stress? ______

______

Safety Hazards in the Sociocultural Environment

What is the extent of crime in the area? ______

What types of crime are involved? ______

______

What is the response time for police personnel? ______

Do area residents take an active part in crime prevention? ______

What is the extent of intergroup conflict in the area? ______

______

Is there tension between racial or ethnic groups in the area? ______

Is there gang violence in the area? ______

What is the extent of family violence in the area? ______

What is the response of protective services personnel to episodes of family violence? ______

______

What is the extent of drug and alcohol use/abuse in the area? ______

______

Are drug dealers a problem in the area? ______

What is the extent of drug-related crime in the area? ______

Disaster Potential

What is the potential for flooding? ______

What is the potential for earthquakes? ______

What is the potential for brushfires or forest fires? ____________________

What is the potential for toxic exposures? ____________________

What is the potential for explosions? ____________________

What is the potential for severe weather events? ____________________

Is there a community disaster plan? _______ If so, are area residents aware of the plan? ____________

Neighborhood/Community Safety Problems Identified

1. ____________________
2. ____________________
3. ____________________
4. ____________________
5. ____________________

Nursing Interventions to Address Safety Problems

1. ____________________
2. ____________________
3. ____________________
4. ____________________
5. ____________________

Expected Outcomes of Nursing Interventions

1. ____________________
2. ____________________
3. ____________________
4. ____________________
5. ____________________

Evaluation of Intervention Outcomes

1. ____________________
2. ____________________
3. ____________________
4. ____________________
5. ____________________

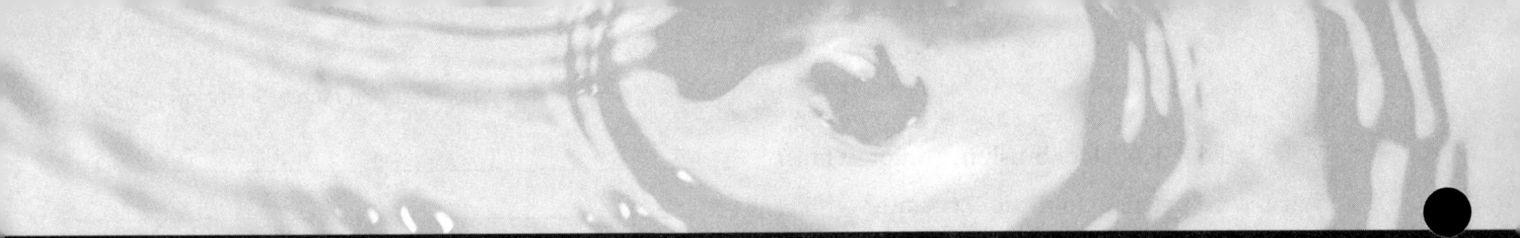

POPULATION HEALTH ASSESSMENT AND INTERVENTION GUIDE

Description: This tool is designed to assist the community health nurse to identify health problems exhibited by communities or population groups. The assessment component of the tool is based on the six dimensions of health addressed in the dimensions model, and the community health nurse is prompted to obtain information on factors in the biophysical, psychological, physical environmental, sociocultural, behavioral, and health system dimensions as they affect community health status. The tool also provides guidance for the development of community nursing diagnoses and for planning, implementing, and evaluating interventions to address identified community health problems.

Appropriate populations: Geopolitical communities or jurisdictions. May also be applied, with modification, to specific target populations within or across geopolitical jurisdictions.

Data sources and data collection strategies: Data collection strategies usually need to be quite varied and may include review of records of community government agencies (including those from local health departments), health care institutions and agencies, schools, chambers of commerce, and so on, as well as interviews with key individuals in these and other organizations. Other strategies for obtaining community assessment information include interviews or surveys of community residents, review of local historical materials, participation in the activities of local groups, review of the telephone directory and other local directories listing service agencies, review of area maps, and walking or driving through the community to make personal observations. Generally speaking, the magnitude and complexity of a community assessment suggest that data collection is more effectively handled by a group of people rather than a single community health nurse. The community health nurse, however, may initiate the assessment process and coordinate data collection activities, in addition to obtaining information him- or herself. The community health nurse should also be actively involved in analysis, interpretation, and dissemination of community assessment findings and in planning programs to address identified community health needs.

Use of information: Information gleaned from the community assessment is used to develop community nursing diagnoses that describe health risks/problems in the community and the resources available within the community for dealing with these risks and problems. From the community nursing diagnoses, planning groups can begin to design community-based interventions to address health concerns. Again, this requires active participation of multiple individuals and agencies in the community and is not an activity that the community health nurse is likely to perform as an independent individual. As noted earlier, however, community health nurses should be actively involved in the planning, implementation, and evaluation of community health programs.

POPULATION HEALTH ASSESSMENT AND INTERVENTION GUIDE

Assessment

Biophysical Considerations

Births (*annual rate, extent of illegitimacy, abortion*): ______________________________

____

Composition of population:

Age	Total	Male	Female	White	African American	Latino Asian	Native American	Other
<1 year								
1–5 years								
6–12 years								
13–20 years								
21–30 years								
31–50 years								
51–65 years								
66–80 years								
>80 years								

Mortality rates (*overall, age-specific, cause-specific*): ______________________________

____

Morbidity:

Disease	Incidence	Prevalence	Disease	Incidence	Prevalence

How do morbidity and mortality rates compare with those of previous years? ______________________________

____

With state and national rates? ______________________________

____

What is the immunization status of the population? ______________________________

____

Are there special immunization issues in the population? ______________________________

____

Psychological Considerations

Future prospects for the community: ____________________

____

Significant events in community history: ____________________

____

Interaction of groups within the community (*racial tension, etc.*): ____________________

____

Protective services (*adequacy, local crime rate, insurance rates*): ____________________

____

Communication network (*media, informal channels, links to outside world*): ____________________

____

Sources of stress in the community: ____________________

____

Extent of mental illness in the community: ____________________

____

Physical Environmental Considerations

Community location (*boundaries, urban/rural*): ____________________

____

Size and density: ____________________

____

Prominent topographical features: ____________________

____

Housing (*type, condition, adequacy, number of persons per dwelling, sanitation*): ____________________

____

Safety hazards present in the environment: ____________________

____

Source of community water supply: ____________________

____

Sewage and waste disposal: ____________________

____

Nuisance factors: ____________________

____

Potential for disaster: ____________________

____

Sociocultural Considerations

Government (*type, effectiveness, community officials*): ______________________________

____

Unofficial leaders (*significant informants*): ______________________________

____

Political affiliations and level of political involvement of community members: ______________

____

Status of minority groups (*influence, length of residence*): ______________________________

____

Languages spoken by community members: ______________________________

____

Community income levels (*poverty, coverage by assistance programs*): ______________________

____

Education (*prevailing levels, attitudes, facilities*): ______________________________

____

Religion (*major affiliations, programs and services, influence on health*): ____________________

____

Culture (*affiliation, influence on health*): ______________________________

____

Employment level: ______________________________

____

Transportation (*type, availability, cost, adequacy*): ______________________________

____

Shopping facilities (*type, availability, cost, use*): ______________________________

____

Social services (*type, availability, adequacy, use*): ______________________________

____

Primary occupations of community members: ______________________________

____

Major employers (*occupational health programs*): ______________________________

____

Occupational hazards: ______________________________

____

Behavioral Considerations

Consumption Patterns

Nutrition (*general levels, preferences, preparation, special needs, prevalence of anemia, obesity*): ______________________

____

Alcohol (*consumption patterns, extent of abuse*): ______________________

____

Drug use (*licit and illicit*): ______________________

____

Tobacco use (*extent, cessation program availability*): ______________________

____

Exercise (*extent, type, opportunity*): ______________________

____

Leisure Activities

Primary leisure activities of community members: ______________________

____

Recreational facilities (*availability, adequacy, cost*): ______________________

____

Health hazards posed by recreation: ______________________

____

Other Behaviors

Use of safety devices (*seatbelts, helmets, child car seats, etc.*): ______________________

____

Contraceptive use: ______________________

____

Health System Considerations

Community attitudes toward health and health services (*definitions, support of services*): ______________________

____

Health services and resources (*type, availability, cost, adequacy, utilization*): ______________________

____

Prenatal care (*availability, use*): ______________________

____

Emergency services (*availability, adequacy*): ______________________

____

Health education services (*availability, adequacy*): ______________________

____

Health care financing (*extent of insurance coverage, Medicaid, Medicare, tax support*): ______________________

____

Diagnosis

Biophysical Diagnoses

Community Health Need/Risk	Need-Service Match/Mismatch

Psychological Diagnoses

Community Health Need/Risk	Need-Service Match/Mismatch

Physical Environmental Diagnoses

Community Health Need/Risk	Need-Service Match/Mismatch

Sociocultural Diagnoses

Community Health Need/Risk	Need-Service Match/Mismatch

Behavioral Diagnoses

Community Health Need/Risk	Need-Service Match/Mismatch

Health system Diagnoses

Community Health Need/Risk	Need-Service Match/Mismatch

Planning

Planned Interventions	Outcome Objectives

Implementation

Intervention	Responsible Party/Expected Completion Date	Status

Evaluation

Expected Outcome	Status (Met/Unmet)	Supporting Evidence

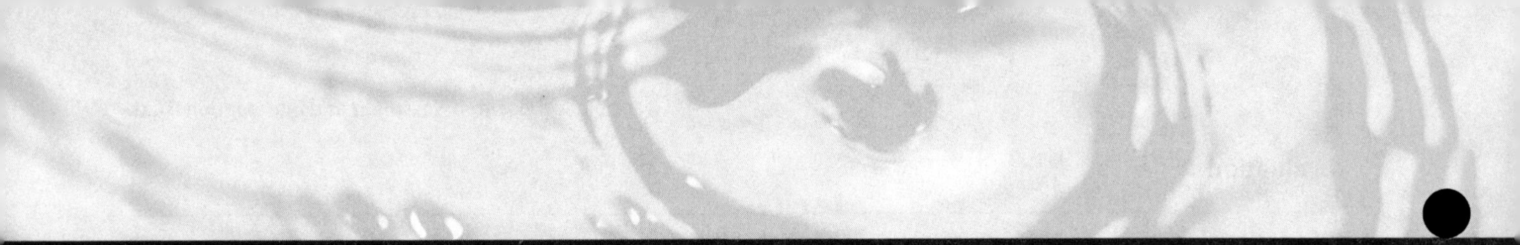

HOME SAFETY INVENTORY—CHILDREN AND ADOLESCENTS

Description: The tool presented here is designed to assist the community health nurse to identify safety hazards in the home.

Appropriate populations: The tool is designed specifically for use with children and adolescents, but can be modified for use with other clients and population groups. For example, the *Home Safety Inventory—Children and Adolescents* could be used to assess environmental safety in childcare or school settings. Many of the items are also relevant to home safety for all clients whatever their age or health status and can be used to identify general safety hazards present in the home or other settings.

Data sources and data collection strategies: Information on areas addressed by the *Home Safety Inventory* can be obtained by interviews with parents, child caretakers, or other family members or by observation of the home setting.

Use of information: The result of the inventory can be used to educate parents or families regarding home safety issues and to motivate changes in environmental conditions to promote safety in the home. The inventories can also be completed by groups of people and the results used to initiate home safety education or public policies to promote home safety.

HOME SAFETY INVENTORY—CHILDREN AND ADOLESCENTS

Age	Safety Consideration	Yes	No
Infant	1. Safe sleeping arrangements made for infant?	❑	❑
	2. Parents aware of bathing safety (not leaving child unattended, water temperature)?	❑	❑
	3. No loose parts on toys?	❑	❑
	4. Approved car restraint used consistently?	❑	❑
	5. Family avoids leaving infant or infant seat on elevated surfaces?	❑	❑
	6. Infant restraint straps consistently used in infant seat, stroller, high chair, car seat?	❑	❑
	7. Small objects kept out of reach?	❑	❑
Toddler/preschool child	1. Poisons, sharp objects, etc., kept locked away?	❑	❑
	2. Poisonous substances stored in appropriate containers?	❑	❑
	3. Childproof lids correctly placed on medications and other toxins?	❑	❑
	4. Medications stored in locked area?	❑	❑
	5. Poison control center number in visible location?	❑	❑
	6. Gates/barriers placed on stairs?	❑	❑
	7. Safety locks present on doors and upstairs windows?	❑	❑
	8. Child closely supervised at play?	❑	❑
	9. Child supervised at all times during bath?	❑	❑
	10. Toys have no small parts?	❑	❑
	11. Electrical outlets covered?	❑	❑
	12. No electrical cords left dangling?	❑	❑
	13. Pots and pans placed toward back of stove with handles turned toward rear?	❑	❑
	14. Play equipment in good repair?	❑	❑
	15. Outdoor play area is fenced and gates locked?	❑	❑
	16. Outdoor play area has resilient surface?	❑	❑
	17. No poisonous plants present in home or yard?	❑	❑
	18. Car seat belt and booster seat used consistently?	❑	❑
	19. Caution used and taught in crossing streets?	❑	❑
School-aged child	1. Child supervised in sports and outdoor play?	❑	❑
	2. Play equipment free of safety hazards?	❑	❑
	3. Outdoor play area floored with sand, shavings, or wood chips?	❑	❑
	4. Firearms kept locked with key inaccessible?	❑	❑
	5. Bicycle helmet worn consistently?	❑	❑
	6. Children taught not to open door to strangers?	❑	❑
	7. Car seat belt used consistently?	❑	❑
Adolescent	1. Firearms safety taught?	❑	❑
	2. Firearms stored unloaded with safety lock on?	❑	❑
	3. Teen cautioned not to admit being home alone?	❑	❑
	4. Car seat belt used consistently?	❑	❑

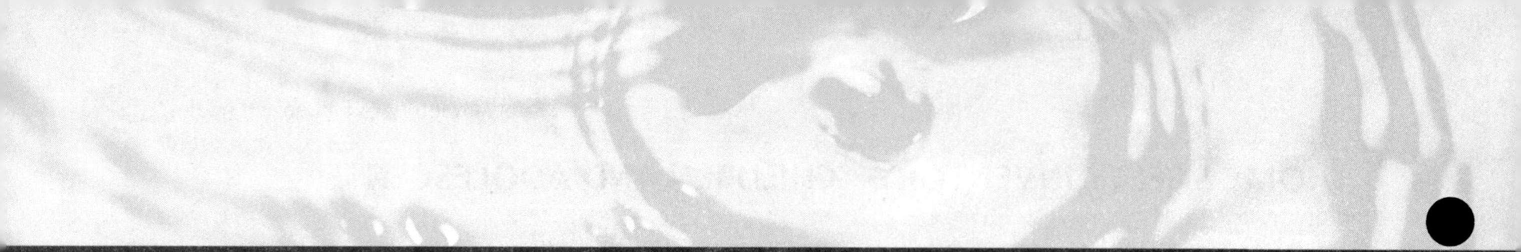

CHILD AND ADOLESCENT HEALTH ASSESSMENT AND INTERVENTION GUIDE

Description: This assessment guide is intended to assist the community health nurse to assess the health status of children and adolescents. The nurse is assisted to identify nursing diagnoses and to plan, implement, and evaluate nursing interventions to promote child and adolescent health and to resolve existing health problems. The assessment component of the tool is based on the epidemiologic perspective of the six dimensions of health.

Appropriate populations: Children from birth through adolescence.

Data sources and data collection strategies: Information regarding the child's or adolescent's health history may be obtained in interviews with parents or other knowledgeable caretakers or from older children themselves. Other sources of information include observations by the nurse and the findings of physical examinations and screening tests. Development may be assessed using a variety of age-appropriate developmental assessment tools (e.g., the Denver II for children from birth to 6 years of age). Parents may also be asked to complete a nutritional diary to provide information on child nutrition.

Use of information: Information obtained using the assessment tool is used to derive both problem-focused and wellness diagnoses. Emphasis is given to using assessment data to design interventions for promoting health and preventing illness as well as resolving existing problems. Special consideration should be given to providing parents with anticipatory guidance concerning their children's development.

CHILD AND ADOLESCENT HEALTH ASSESSMENT AND INTERVENTION GUIDE

Name: ______________________________ Phone: ______________

Address: ____

Guardian: ____________________ Relationship to child/adolescent: __________

Assessment

Biophysical Considerations

Maturation and Aging/Genetic Inheritance

Age: ________ Date of birth: __________ Gender: _______ Race/ethnic group: ____________

Birth weight and length: ______________________________

Pattern of growth (*compared with norms and previous pattern*): ______________________

Accomplishment of developmental milestones (*DDST or other appropriate test*): ____________

Parental knowledge of child development and its implications: ______________________

Significant family health history (*include genogram*): ______________________

Physiologic Function

Significant events during pregnancy: ______________________

Congenital defects: ______________________

Current acute or chronic illnesses (*describe problem, status, treatment, if any*): ____________

Current signs or symptoms of physical health problems: ______________________

Areas of physical disability or limitation of function: ______________________

Significant past illnesses, injuries, hospitalizations (*what, when, outcomes*): ____________

Review of Systems

Head (*headache* [how often, quality, treatment outcome], *syncope, trauma*): ____________

Eyes (*vision problems, burning eyes, glasses, last eye exam, blocked tear duct, discharge, tearing, itching*): ________

Ears (*difficulty hearing, discharge, earache, frequent otitis*): ______________________________

____

Mouth and throat (*sore throat, lesions, toothache, caries, last dental visit*): ______________________________

____

Respiratory system (*frequent colds, nosebleeds, cough, pneumonia, asthma, shortness of breath, sinusitis, hay fever*): ______

____

Cardiovascular system (*heart problems, hypertension, chest pain, cyanosis* [especially when crying or physically active], *shortness of breath, murmurs, edema*): ______________________________

____

Gastrointestinal system (*nausea, vomiting, diarrhea, constipation, flatulence, abdominal pain, loss of appetite, weight loss or gain, rectal pain or bleeding, quality of stool, frequency*): ______________________________

____

Urinary tract (*dysuria, urinary frequency, urgency, nocturia, difficulty voiding, urinary retention, CVA pain, odor, strength of urinary stream, number of wet diapers in infant*): ______________________________

____

Reproductive system (*vaginal or penile discharge, development of secondary sex characteristics, menarche, dysmenorrhea, wet dreams, extent of sex education, extent of sexual activity, age at sexual debut, history of STD*): ______________

____

____

Musculoskeletal system (*joint pain; swelling; tremor; history of trauma; history of fracture, sprain, or strain; muscle weakness*): ______________________________

____

Integumentary system (*eczema, diaper rash, lesions* [describe character, locale, color], *changes in skin color, itching, hair loss, discoloration or pitting of nails, clubbing of nails, birthmarks, swollen glands, piercing, tattoos*): ______________

____

Hematopoietic system (*anemia, bleeding tendencies, bruise easily, transfusions* [when, why]): ______________

____

Immunization status (*up-to-date for age*): ______________________________

____

Physical Examination

Height, weight, head and chest circumference: ______________________________

____

Vital signs (*T, P, R, B/P*): ______________________________

____

General appearance (*posture, gait, deformities, hygiene*): ______________________________

____

Skin (*diaper rash, eczema, acne, milia, bruises, burns, hygiene, tattoos*): ________________________________

____

Head and neck (*lymph nodes, face*): ____

____

Eyes (*ability to focus and follow objects*): ____

____

Ears (*ability to localize sound*): ____

____

Nose and sinuses: ____

____

Mouth and throat (*monilial patches, number of teeth, dental hygiene, caries*): _______________

____

Chest:

Breast examination (*newborn engorgement, precocious puberty, normal breast development, gynecomastia*): ________

____

Heart (*murmurs, split heart sounds*): ____

____

Lungs: ____

____

Abdomen: ____

____

Genitalia (*undescended testes, vaginal tears, discharge, imperforate anus, secondary sex characteristics*): ____________

____

Musculoskeletal system (*symmetry of extremities, spina bifida, scoliosis, congenital hip dislocation, muscle strength*): ____

____

____

Nervous system (*cranial nerves, DTRs, temperature, kinesthetic sense, tremor, newborn reflexes*): ______________

____

Screening test results (*PKU, T4, hematocrit, sickle cell, serum lead, TB, urinalysis, STDs, pregnancy, as appropriate*):

____

____

Psychological Considerations

Reactivity patterns and parental responses: ____

____

Parental expectations (*appropriateness*): ____

____

Gender socialization and effects on health: ____

Discipline (*type, consistency, appropriateness*): ______

Parental coping skills: ______

Parent–child interactions: ______

Self-image: ______

Emotional state or mood (*usual, recent changes*): ______

Evidence of abuse or neglect: ______

Recent experience of significant loss (*death, divorce, move*): ______

Evidence of mental health problem: ______

Suicide ideation: ______

Level of social or parental pressure to perform: ______

Physical Environmental Considerations

Where does the client live? ______

Is there adequate space and privacy in the home? ______

Are safety hazards present in the home? (*See Home Safety Inventory*) ______

Extent of age-appropriate child-proofing of home: ______

Presence of weapons in the home: ______

Are there pets in the home? (*What kind? How many? Inside or outside?*) ______

What is the neighborhood like? (*safety, pollutants, etc.*) ______

What pollutants are present in the environment? (*secondhand smoke*) ______

What health effects do pollutants have? ______

Sociocultural Considerations

Education (*grade, performance*): ______

Interaction with peers: ______

Interaction with others: ______

Cultural-child rearing attitudes/practices: ______

Parental education level: ______

Language spoken in the home: ______

Intergenerational conflict: ______

Childcare outside the home (*where, by whom, adequacy*): ______

Parental employment and effects on child/adolescent: ______

Family responsibilities/expectations: ______

Employment of child or adolescent (*type, hours, health effects*): ______

Behavioral Considerations

Consumption Patterns

Infant (*formula, breast, amount, formula preparation, feeding and burping techniques*): ______

Other age groups (*well-balanced diet, amount of "junk food," food allergies*): ______

Parental knowledge of nutrition needs: ______

Exposure to drugs/alcohol/tobacco smoke: ______

Use of alcohol/tobacco/other drugs: ______

Rest and Exercise

Sleep patterns: ______

Type and amount of exercise: ______

Use of safety precautions, equipment: ______

Other

Sexual activity (*frequency, use of contraceptives, condoms, sexual practices/orientation*): ______

Use of seat belts, other safety devices: ______

Extent of safety education: ___

Cultural practice of FGM: ___

Chronic disease self-care (*need, knowledge, efficacy*): ___

___

Risk-taking behavior: ___

Health System Considerations

Use of primary prevention services (*general and dental*): ___

___

Source of illness care: ___

___

Parental knowledge of illness care and need for medical assistance: ___

___

Availability of needed health care services: ___

Use of available health care services: ___

Financing of health care services (*insurance, adequacy*): ___

Barriers to health care services: ___

(For guidelines related to nursing diagnoses, planning, implementation, and evaluation of interventions for children and adolescents use pages 35–36 of the *Family Health Assessment and Intervention Guide.*)

NUTRITIONAL ASSESSMENT OF CHILDREN AND ADOLESCENTS

Age Group	Assessment Questions	Yes	No
Infant (birth–1 year)	Is the child breast- or bottle-fed? ________________		
	If breast-fed:		
	How often does the child nurse? ________________		
	How long does the child nurse? ________________		
	Does mother alternate breasts?	❑	❑
	Is mother's nutritional intake adequate?	❑	❑
	Does the child seem satisfied?	❑	❑
	If bottle-fed:		
	How often does the baby eat? ________________		
	How much formula is consumed in 24 hours? ____________		
	What type of formula is used? ________________		
	Is it iron-fortified?	❑	❑
	Do parents prepare formula correctly?	❑	❑
	Do parents use appropriate feeding techniques (e.g., not propping the bottle)?	❑	❑
	Does the infant tolerate the formula well?	❑	❑
	Is the infant gaining weight?	❑	❑
	At what point did parents introduce solids? ______________		
	How much solid food does the baby eat? ______________		
	Do parents use individual foods rather than less nutritious combination foods (such as vegetable and beef combinations)?	❑	❑
	Is one new food introduced at a time? Over several days?	❑	❑
	Has the child started eating table food? (This usually occurs at about 9 months of age.)	❑	❑
	Is the child weaned from the bottle by 1 year?	❑	❑
Toddler and preschool child (2–5 years)	What foods is the child eating? ________________________________		
	How much food is the child eating? ________________________________		
	Is fluid intake adequate?	❑	❑
	Is the child's diet well balanced?	❑	❑
	Is the child eating the recommended number of daily servings of fruits, vegetables, and grains?	❑	❑
	Is the child's diet low in saturated fat and sodium?	❑	❑
	Is the child's calcium and iron intake adequate?	❑	❑
	Are finger foods and variety encouraged?	❑	❑
	Are any snacks provided nutritious?	❑	❑
	Is the child given small portions initially and allowed to ask for more to enhance independence?	❑	❑
	Is the child's growth pattern normal for his or her age?	❑	❑

Age Group	Assessment Questions	Yes	No
School-aged child (6–12 years)	Is the child's diet well balanced?	❑	❑
	Are junk food and sodas avoided?	❑	❑
	Are snacks nutritious?	❑	❑
	Is the child eating the recommended number of daily servings of fruits, vegetables, and grains?	❑	❑
	Is the child's diet low in saturated fat and sodium?	❑	❑
	Is the child's calcium and iron intake adequate?	❑	❑
	How much does the child eat? ______________________________		
	Is the child overweight or underweight?	❑	❑
	Is the child's weight within normal limits for his or her age?	❑	❑
Adolescent (13–18 years)	Is the adolescent's diet well balanced?	❑	❑
	Are junk food and sodas avoided?	❑	❑
	Are snacks nutritious?	❑	❑
	Is the adolescent eating the recommended number of daily servings of fruits, vegetables, and grains?	❑	❑
	Is the adolescent's diet low in saturated fat and sodium?	❑	❑
	Is the adolescent's protein and calcium intake adequate to accommodate growth spurts?	❑	❑
	Is iron intake sufficient to accommodate blood loss in menstruating girls?	❑	❑
	How much does the adolescent eat?______________________		
	Is the adolescent overweight or underweight?	❑	❑
	Is the adolescent's weight within normal limits for his or her height?	❑	❑
	Does the adolescent engage in fad dieting?	❑	❑
	Does the adolescent engage in binging or purging?	❑	❑
	Is the adolescent excessively concerned about body size?	❑	❑
	Is the adolescent consuming excessive caffeine?	❑	❑
	Is the adolescent consuming alcohol?	❑	❑

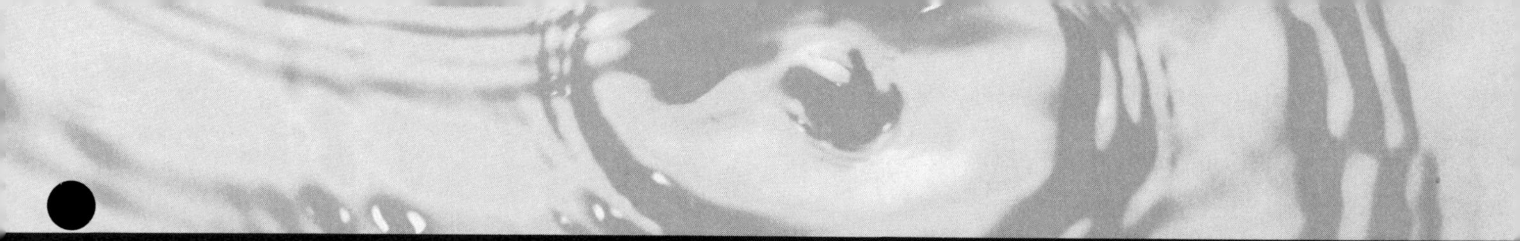

CHILD AND ADOLESCENT DEVELOPMENT INVENTORY

Age	Criterion	Yes	No
Birth–1 month	Newborn reflexes intact?	❑	❑
	Head lag present?	❑	❑
	Follows objects to midline with eyes?	❑	❑
	Responds to noise?	❑	❑
	Regards human face?	❑	❑
	Quiets when picked up?	❑	❑
1–2 months	Follows objects 180° with eyes?	❑	❑
	Holds head up in prone position?	❑	❑
	Head erect and bobbing when supported in sitting position?	❑	❑
	Vocalizes other than crying?	❑	❑
	Smiles responsively?	❑	❑
2–4 months	Newborn reflexes diminishing?	❑	❑
	Sits well with support?	❑	❑
	Rolls from side to side?	❑	❑
	Grasps rattle?	❑	❑
	Laughs aloud?	❑	❑
	Initiates smiles?	❑	❑
	Enjoys play activity?	❑	❑
4–6 months	Reaches for and gets objects?	❑	❑
	Puts objects in mouth?	❑	❑
	Rolls over completely?	❑	❑
	Supports own weight when standing?	❑	❑
	First teeth erupting?	❑	❑
	Turns to voice?	❑	❑
	Shows beginning stranger anxiety?	❑	❑
	Shows strong attachment to primary caretaker?	❑	❑
6–9 months	Sits alone?	❑	❑
	Bounces?	❑	❑
	Stands holding on?	❑	❑
	Demonstrates thumb-finger grasp?	❑	❑
	Says "mama" or "dada"?	❑	❑
	Plays peek-a-boo and patty cake?	❑	❑
	Imitates speech sounds?	❑	❑
9–12 months	Pulls to stand?	❑	❑
	Creeps or crawls?	❑	❑
	Walks holding on?	❑	❑
	Sits from standing position?	❑	❑
	Drinks from cup with help?	❑	❑
	Gives toy on request?	❑	❑
	Speaks two to three words?	❑	❑
	Gives affection?	❑	❑
	Indicates wants?	❑	❑
12–18 months	Scribbles?	❑	❑
	Points to one or more body parts?	❑	❑
	Uses a spoon?	❑	❑

Age	Criterion	Yes	No
	Climbs and runs?	☐	☐
	Plays ball?	☐	☐
	Beginning bowel training?	☐	☐
	Likes to be read to?	☐	☐
	Has 10-word vocabulary?	☐	☐
18–24 months	Opens doors?	☐	☐
	Turns on faucets?	☐	☐
	Throws or kicks a ball?	☐	☐
	Walks up and down stairs alone?	☐	☐
	Daytime bowel and bladder control established?	☐	☐
	Engages in parallel play?	☐	☐
	Uses two- to three-word sentences?	☐	☐
	Imitates household tasks?	☐	☐
2–3 years	Dresses with help?	☐	☐
	Rides a tricycle?	☐	☐
	Washes and dries hands?	☐	☐
	Separates easily from primary caretaker?	☐	☐
	Uses pronouns?	☐	☐
	Perceives danger?	☐	☐
	Understands sharing and taking turns?	☐	☐
3–5 years	Dresses with decreasing supervision?	☐	☐
	Hops on one foot?	☐	☐
	Catches bounced ball?	☐	☐
	Demonstrates heel-to-toe walk?	☐	☐
	Gives whole name?	☐	☐
	Recognizes three colors?	☐	☐
	Draws a person with more than six parts?	☐	☐
	Tells a story?	☐	☐
	Operates from rules?	☐	☐
5–10 years	Physical growth slowing?	☐	☐
	Demonstrates increasing motor coordination?	☐	☐
	Beginning peer identification?	☐	☐
	Forms friendships?	☐	☐
	Learning more rules?	☐	☐
	Beginning gender identification?	☐	☐
	Increasing use of language to convey ideas?	☐	☐
	Beginning to understand cause and effect?	☐	☐
11–14 years	Beginning pubertal changes?	☐	☐
	Demonstrates gawkiness?	☐	☐
	Demonstrates importance of peer group conformity?	☐	☐
	Displays strong identification with sexmates?	☐	☐
	Learning his or her role in heterosexual relationships?	☐	☐
	Beginning to establish an identity?	☐	☐
	Engages in more abstract thought?	☐	☐
	Displays negative attitude toward family?	☐	☐
15–18 years	Has completed pubertal changes and adolescent growth spurt?	☐	☐
	Is more coordinated in handling the "new" body?	☐	☐
	Has developed an independent identity?	☐	☐
	Has established relationships with members of the opposite gender?	☐	☐
	Has adopted an adult value set?	☐	☐
	Is moving away from family relationships?	☐	☐
	Has identified possible career options or goals?	☐	☐

SAFETY EDUCATION INVENTORY FOR CHILDREN AND ADOLESCENTS

Age	Safety Education Element Addressed?	Yes	No
Infant (birth–1year)	Not leaving child unattended on elevated surfaces or in bath?	❑	❑
	Use of car seat restraint?	❑	❑
	Use of safety straps in high chairs, strollers, swings, infant seats, etc.?	❑	❑
	Use of flame-retardant sleepwear?	❑	❑
	Crib safety: Narrow spaces between slats, bumper pads, no plastic coverings, nontoxic paint, no soft pillows?	❑	❑
	Toy safety: No sharp edges or small parts, no long strings, no loose parts, siblings' toys out of reach?	❑	❑
Toddler (1–3 years)	Not leaving child unattended in pool, bath, or car?	❑	❑
	Use of car seat restraint?	❑	❑
	Adequate adult supervision at all times?	❑	❑
	Home safety: Outlet covers, sharp and poisonous objects locked away, medications out of reach, child-resistant containers used, gated stairs, cupboard and door latches installed, bathroom doors closed, no dangling electrical cords?	❑	❑
	Play equipment: Age-appropriate and in good repair, on an appropriate surface?	❑	❑
	Toy safety: Age-appropriate toys, no small parts?	❑	❑
	Fenced yard/swimming pool?	❑	❑
Preschool child (3–6 years)	Use of booster seat in vehicle?	❑	❑
	Adequate adult supervision?	❑	❑
	Home safety: Outlet covers, sharp and poisonous objects locked away, medications out of reach, child-resistant containers used, gated stairs, cupboard and door latches installed, bathroom doors closed, no dangling electrical cords?	❑	❑
	Play equipment: Age-appropriate and in good repair, on an appropriate surface?	❑	❑
	Toy safety: Age-appropriate toys, no small parts, adult supervision with potentially hazardous toys?	❑	❑
	Fenced yard/swimming pool?	❑	❑
	Safety practices: Education regarding interaction with strangers, crossing the street, fire safety, water safety?	❑	❑
School-age child (6–12 years)	Use of booster seat/adult seat belt based on height and weight?	❑	❑
	Sports safety: Age-appropriate sports, use of safety equipment, adequate adult supervision?	❑	❑
	Firearms: Locked separately from ammunition?	❑	❑
	Safety practices: Education regarding stranger interactions, caring for self at home, sports, bicycling and helmet use, water safety, use of medications, swimming instruction?	❑	❑

Age	Safety Education Element Addressed?	Yes	No
Adolescent (13–18 years)	Safe driving?	❑	❑
	Use of seat belts?	❑	❑
	Sports safety: Age-appropriate sports, use of safety equipment, adequate adult supervision?	❑	❑
	Safety practices: Education regarding use of firearms, caring for self and others at home, use of medications, dangerous situations (e.g., alcohol or other drugs and driving, fighting), stranger interactions?	❑	❑
	Sexuality: Abstinence, safe sexual practices?	❑	❑
	Use of drugs and alcohol?	❑	❑

HEALTH ASSESSMENT AND INTERVENTION GUIDE—ADULT WOMAN

Description: This assessment guide is intended to assist the community health nurse to assess the health needs of adult women and to direct the planning, implementation, and evaluation of nursing interventions to meet identified needs. The assessment component of the tool is based on the six dimensions of health in the dimensions model of community health nursing.

Appropriate populations: May be used with young and middle adult female clients. Assessment of adolescent girls would employ the *Child and Adolescent Health Assessment and Intervention Guide* on pages 52–58. Community health nurses assessing the needs of older women should use the *Health Assessment and Intervention Guide—Older Adult* on pages 89–94.

Data sources and data collection strategies: Information required for assessing adult women is usually obtained from client interviews. Additional data may be obtained from health records, laboratory test results, and the observations of the nurse. For mentally incompetent clients, data may be obtained from significant others.

Use of information: The information gleaned from the assessment is used by the community health nurse to make nursing diagnoses and to plan, implement, and evaluate nursing care to address women's health needs.

HEALTH ASSESSMENT AND INTERVENTION GUIDE—ADULT WOMAN

Client's name: ______________________________ Phone: ______________

Address: ____

Assessment

Biophysical Considerations

Maturation and Aging/Genetic Inheritance

Age: ______________ Date of birth: ______________ Race/ethnic group: ______________

Accomplishment of adult developmental tasks: ______________________________

____

Significant family health history (*include genogram*): ______________________________

____

Physiologic Function

Current acute or chronic illnesses (*describe problem, status, treatment, if any*): ______________

____

Current signs or symptoms of physical health problems: ______________________________

____

Areas of physical disability or limitation of function: ______________________________

____

Significant past illnesses, surgery, injuries, hospitalizations (*what, when, outcomes*): ______________

____

Current pregnancy or pregnancy-related concerns: ______________________________

____

Review of Systems

Head (*headache* [how often, quality, treatment outcome], *syncope, trauma*): ______________

____

Eyes (*vision problems, burning eyes, glasses, last eye exam, blocked tear duct, discharge, tearing, itching*): ______________

____

Ears (*difficulty hearing, discharge, earache*): ______________________________

____

Mouth and throat (*sore throat, lesions, toothache, caries, last dental visit*): ______________

____

Respiratory system (*frequent colds, nosebleeds, cough, pneumonia, asthma, shortness of breath, sinusitis, hay fever*): ______________

____

____

Cardiovascular system (*heart problems, hypertension, chest pain, cyanosis, shortness of breath, murmurs, edema*): ______________

____

Gastrointestinal system (*nausea, vomiting, diarrhea, constipation, flatulence, abdominal pain, loss of appetite, weight loss or gain, rectal pain or bleeding*): ______

______

Urinary tract (*dysuria, urinary frequency, urgency, nocturia, difficulty voiding, urinary retention, CVA pain*): ______

______

______

Reproductive system (*breast lumps, changes in breast contour, breast discharge, last mammogram, dysmenorrhea, irregular menses, excessively heavy periods, edema of labia or vulva, vaginal discharge* [color, character, odor], *dyspareunia, PMS, last pap smear, sexual activity, use of oral or other contraceptives, condom use, sexual satisfaction, number of sexual partners, sexual orientation, history of STDs, history of FGM*): ______

______

______

______

LMP: ______ Age at menarche: ______

Pregnancy history/outcomes: ______

______

______

Musculoskeletal system (*joint pain, swelling, tremor, history of trauma, muscle weakness, osteoporosis, calcium intake, history of fractures*): ______

______

Integumentary system (*lesions* [describe character, locale, color], *changes in skin color, itching, hair loss, discoloration or pitting of nails, birthmarks, swollen glands*): ______

______

Neurological system (*seizures, ataxia, tics, tremors, paralysis*): ______

______

Hematopoietic system (*anemia, bleeding tendencies, bruise easily, transfusions* [when, why]): ______

______

Immunologic system (*frequent infections, HIV infection, use of immunosuppressives*): ______

______

Immunization status: ______

Physical Examination

Height and weight: ______

Vital signs (*T, P, R, B/P*): ______

General appearance (*posture, gait, deformities, hygiene*): ______

______

Skin (*include hair and nails*): ______

______

Head and neck (*lymph nodes, face*): ______

______

Eyes: ______

Ears: ______

Nose and sinuses: ______

Mouth and throat (*lips, gums, palate, pharynx, tongue, teeth*): ______

______

Chest:

Breast examination: ______

Heart: ______

Lungs: ______

Abdomen: ______

Genitalia (*including anus and rectum, ovaries, evidence of FGM*): ______

______

Musculoskeletal system (*extremities, spine, joints, muscles*): ______

______

Nervous system (*cranial nerves, DTRs, temperature, kinesthetic sense*): ______

______

Results of screening and other tests: ______

______

______

Psychological Considerations

Self-image, level of self-esteem: ______

______

History of mental illness: ______

______

Emotional mood or state (*current and recent changes*): ______

______

Level of orientation: ______

______

Coping (*strategies used, effectiveness*): ______

______

Recent experience of significant loss (*death, divorce, relocation, effects*): ______

______

Suicide ideation: ______

______

Communication with others (*extent, adequacy*): ______

______

Interpersonal relationships (*extent, satisfaction*): ______

______

Stress (*sources, coping skills, support*): ____________________

____

Evidence of physical or emotional abuse: ____________________

____

Physical Environmental Considerations

Where does the client live? Is there adequate space and privacy in the home? ____________________

____

Are safety hazards present in the home? In the work setting? ____________________

____

Are there pets in the home? (*What kind? How many? Inside or outside?*) ____________________

____

What is the neighborhood like? (*Safety, pollutants, etc.*) ____________________

____

Sociocultural Considerations

Education (*formal education, health knowledge, special learning needs*): ____________________

____

Income (*source, adequacy, budgeting skills*): ____________________

____

Social support network (*components, adequacy, use, marital status, character of marital relationship*): ____________________

____

Cultural practices influencing health: ____________________

____

Gender socialization and effects on health: ____________________

____

Family relationships and effects on health: ____________________

____

Family responsibilities (*caretaker roles, caretaker burden, other roles*): ____________________

____

Extent of social support for healthy behavior: ____________________

____

Religious affiliation (*importance/influence on health*): ____________________

____

Adequacy of adult role models: ____________________

____

Employment (*current and past, hazards, job change pattern*): ____________________

____

Access to transportation: ____________________

Behavioral Considerations

Consumption Patterns

Usual diet (*meal pattern, preferences, preparation, nutritional adequacy, special needs, cultural restrictions*): ______________

Use of alcohol, tobacco, other drugs: ______________

Use of caffeine: ______________

Use of medications (*type, appropriateness*): ______________

Rest and Exercise

Sleep patterns: ______________

Type and amount of exercise: ______________

Leisure (*type of activity, hazards posed*): ______________

Other

Sexual activity (*frequency, use of contraceptives, condoms, sexual orientation, multiple partners, sexual practices*): ______________

Use of seat belts, other safety devices: ______________

Health System Considerations

Use of primary prevention services (*general and dental*): ______________

Attitudes toward health and health care: ______________

Usual source of health care: ______________

Health care financing (*type, adequacy*): ______________

Barriers to care: ______________

Use of health care services (*appropriateness*): ______________

(For guidelines related to nursing diagnoses, planning, implementation, and evaluation of interventions for women use pages 35–36 of the *Family Health Assessment and Intervention Guide.*)

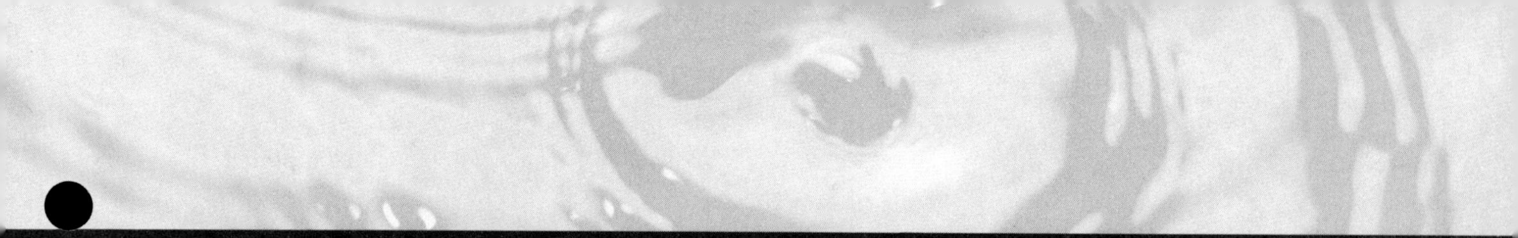

PRENATAL CARE INVENTORY

Intervention	Completed: Yes	Completed: No
Biophysical Considerations		
First trimester		
Obtain past pregnancy history	❑	❑
Identify risks posed by age of mother, if any	❑	❑
Determine prepregnant weight, periodic weight check	❑	❑
Obtain medical history (e.g., HIV infection, TB, diabetes)	❑	❑
Assess for edema and voiding	❑	❑
Address normal discomforts of pregnancy (e.g., nausea, vomiting, constipation, heartburn, urinary frequency, etc.); suggest measures for alleviation of discomforts	❑	❑
Assess for anemia	❑	❑
Check blood pressure on each visit	❑	❑
Encourage loose-fitting clothing and properly fitted shoes	❑	❑
Teach signs of complications of pregnancy	❑	❑
Assess for dental hygiene, problems; encourage dental hygiene; refer as needed for dental problems	❑	❑
Assess for fetal movement	❑	❑
Monitor existing health problems (e.g., diabetes)	❑	❑
Assess risk for congenital problems (e.g., family history, communicable disease exposure, etc.)	❑	❑
Second trimester		
Assess fundal height	❑	❑
Assess fetal heart tones	❑	❑
Check blood pressure regularly	❑	❑
Continue to monitor existing health problems	❑	❑
Monitor for signs of complications	❑	❑
Educate regarding abnormal signs and symptoms (e.g., bleeding)	❑	❑
Educate regarding Braxton-Hicks contractions	❑	❑
Educate for relief of back pain (heels with slight elevation, pelvic rocking, etc.)	❑	❑
Assess fetal movement	❑	❑
Third trimester		
Assess fundal height	❑	❑
Assess fetal heart tones	❑	❑
Check blood pressure regularly	❑	❑
Continue to monitor existing health problems	❑	❑
Assess for lightening	❑	❑
Assess fetal position, movement	❑	❑
Teach signs of labor	❑	❑
Refer for childbirth preparation classes	❑	❑
Psychological Considerations		
First trimester		
Assess feelings regarding pregnancy	❑	❑
Assess for emotional lability, reassure of normality	❑	❑

Intervention	Completed Yes	Completed No
Identify preexisting mental or emotional illness; refer for care as needed	❑	❑
Assess for evidence of abuse; refer for assistance as needed	❑	❑
Second trimester		
Monitor signs of early bonding with baby	❑	❑
Continue to assess for possible abuse	❑	❑
Third trimester		
Assist client to deal with waiting, restlessness	❑	❑
Continue to monitor feelings regarding pregnancy	❑	❑
Continue to assess for possible abuse	❑	❑
Physical Environmental Considerations		
First trimester		
Assess adequacy of living arrangements, space for new baby	❑	❑
Assess safety hazards in home	❑	❑
Assess for presence of pets in home	❑	❑
Assess for secondhand smoke in home	❑	❑
Third trimester		
Assist in planning sleeping arrangements for baby	❑	❑
Assist with reallocation of space among family members, if needed	❑	❑
Assist in planning for pets to promote infant health and safety	❑	❑
Educate regarding effects of secondhand smoke on infant	❑	❑
Sociocultural Considerations		
First trimester		
Assess extent of support system	❑	❑
Assess parental role models	❑	❑
Assess knowledge of childcare	❑	❑
Assess financial status; refer for assistance as needed	❑	❑
Assess cultural beliefs and practices related to pregnancy	❑	❑
Assess relationship with father of child, other family members	❑	❑
Second trimester		
Begin preparation of siblings for new baby	❑	❑
Third trimester		
Assist with obtaining baby items, if needed	❑	❑
Encourage plans for care of other children	❑	❑
Assist with arranging transportation to hospital	❑	❑
Encourage client to explore childcare arrangements if returning to work	❑	❑
Continue preparation of siblings	❑	❑
Assist with development of new roles, reallocation of previous roles	❑	❑
Teach parenting skills as needed	❑	❑
Behavioral Considerations		
First trimester		
Assess diet; educate on nutritional needs in pregnancy as needed	❑	❑
Refer for nutritional supplement program or counseling as needed	❑	❑
Encourage vitamin supplements, iron, etc.	❑	❑
Assess use of tobacco, alcohol, other drugs	❑	❑
Educate regarding effects of perinatal substance exposure as needed	❑	❑
Refer for smoking cessation assistance as needed	❑	❑

Intervention	Completed Yes	Completed No
Refer for assistance with substance use/abuse, if needed	❑	❑
Assess for balance between rest and exercise	❑	❑
Encourage adequate exercise and relaxation	❑	❑
Assess sexual activity; educate regarding alternate positions for comfort	❑	❑
Encourage decision on breast- or bottle-feeding	❑	❑
Second trimester		
Continue to encourage adequate diet, exercise, etc.	❑	❑
Third trimester		
Discuss plans for contraception if desired; educate as needed	❑	❑
Caution against sexual activity late in trimester	❑	❑
Health System Considerations		
First trimester		
Refer for prenatal care if not yet obtained	❑	❑
Refer for financial assistance with prenatal care as needed	❑	❑
Second trimester		
Encourage continued prenatal care	❑	❑
Third trimester		
Encourage continued prenatal care	❑	❑

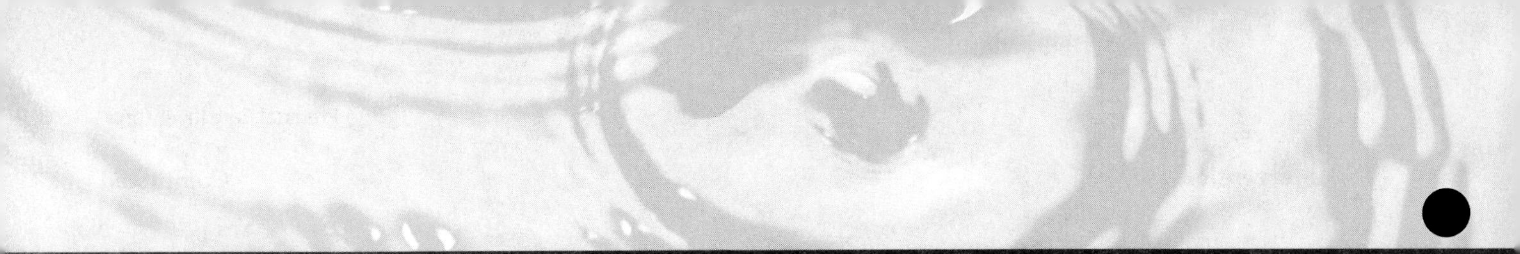

POSTPARTUM/NEWBORN INTERVENTION INVENTORY

Intervention	Completed: Yes	Completed: No
Biophysical Considerations		
Check maternal blood pressure	❑	❑
Check fundal height	❑	❑
Check lochia	❑	❑
Examine breasts for cracks or fissures, engorgement, milk leakage	❑	❑
Check episiotomy	❑	❑
Assess infant growth pattern (height, weight, head/chest circumference)	❑	❑
Assess infant hygiene	❑	❑
Conduct physical examination of newborn	❑	❑
Reassure mother regarding normal newborn variations, molding, etc.	❑	❑
Assess bowel and bladder function (mother and newborn)	❑	❑
Assess infant developmental level	❑	❑
Psychological Considerations		
Assess for postpartum depression	❑	❑
Assess maternal–infant bonding	❑	❑
Assess parental expectations of infant	❑	❑
Assess expectations of self as parent	❑	❑
Assess impact of physical changes on self-image	❑	❑
Encourage client to verbalize regarding labor and delivery experience	❑	❑
Physical Environmental Considerations		
Assess sleeping arrangements for infant	❑	❑
Assess adequacy of living conditions	❑	❑
Assess for presence of pets in home; educate regarding infant safety	❑	❑
Sociocultural Considerations		
Assess impact of infant on family	❑	❑
Assess sibling response to newborn	❑	❑
Assess financial impact of infant	❑	❑
Encourage time alone with other children, if any	❑	❑
Provide assistance with sibling rivalry as needed	❑	❑
Assess ability to cope with role changes	❑	❑
Assist with plans to return to work, as needed (e.g., child-care arrangements)	❑	❑
Assess extent of support system and client's ability to accept help	❑	❑
Assess cultural beliefs and practices related to postpartum/newborn period and potential effects on health	❑	❑
Assess relationship with extended family	❑	❑
Assess relationship with father of child	❑	❑
Refer to mothers' support groups as needed	❑	❑
Behavioral Considerations		
Educate regarding postpartum/breast-feeding diet	❑	❑
Refer for breast-feeding support as needed	❑	❑
Educate regarding infant nutrition	❑	❑

Intervention	Completed Yes	Completed No
Encourage breast-feeding	❑	❑
Observe feeding technique (breast or bottle); educate as needed	❑	❑
Discourage early introduction of foods for infant	❑	❑
Refer for food supplement programs, if needed	❑	❑
Encourage regular exercise	❑	❑
Educate regarding resumption of sexual activity	❑	❑
Assess need for contraceptives; educate or refer as needed	❑	❑
Discuss effects of alcohol, drugs on breast milk	❑	❑
Discuss effects of smoking on newborn, if family members smoke	❑	❑
Refer for smoking cessation assistance if desired	❑	❑
Observe childcare techniques; educate as needed	❑	❑
Educate regarding infant safety practices	❑	❑
Assess infant wake/sleep patterns	❑	❑
Health System Considerations		
Refer for postpartum check if appointment not yet made	❑	❑
Educate regarding infant immunizations	❑	❑
Educate regarding minor illness care	❑	❑
Refer for well child services, immunizations	❑	❑
Refer for contraceptive services as needed	❑	❑

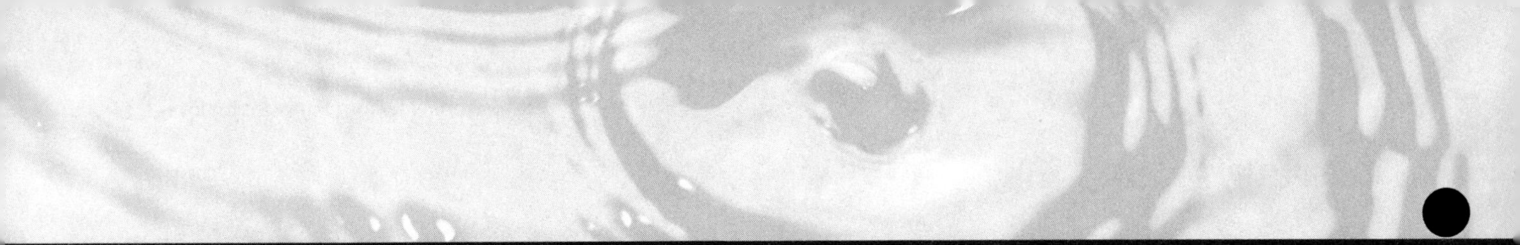

HEALTH ASSESSMENT AND INTERVENTION GUIDE—ADULT MAN

Description: This assessment guide is intended to assist the community health nurse to assess the health needs of adult men and to direct the planning, implementation, and evaluation of nursing interventions to meet identified needs. The assessment component of the tool is based on the six dimensions of health in the dimensions model of community health nursing.

Appropriate populations: May be used with young and middle adult male clients. Assessment of adolescent boys would employ the *Child and Adolescent Health Assessment and Intervention Guide* on pages 52–58. Community health nurses assessing the needs of older men should use the *Health Assessment and Intervention Guide—Older Adult* on pages 89–94.

Data sources and data collection strategies: Information required for assessing adult men is usually obtained from client interviews. Additional data may be obtained from health records, laboratory test results, and the observations of the nurse. For mentally incompetent clients, data may be obtained from significant others.

Use of information: The information gleaned from the assessment is used by the community health nurse to make nursing diagnoses and to plan, implement, and evaluate nursing care to address men's health needs.

HEALTH ASSESSMENT AND INTERVENTION GUIDE—ADULT MAN

Client's name: ______________________________ Phone: ______________

Address: ____

Assessment

Biophysical Considerations

Maturation and Aging/Genetic Inheritance

Age: _______ Date of birth: _______ Race/ethnic group: ______________________

Accomplishment of adult developmental tasks: ______________________________

____

Significant family health history (*include genogram*): ______________________

____

Physiologic Function

Current acute or chronic illnesses (*describe problem, status, treatment, if any*): ______________

____

Current signs or symptoms of physical health problems: ______________________

____

Areas of physical disability or limitation of function: ______________________

____

Significant past illnesses, surgery, injuries, hospitalizations (*what, when, outcomes*): ______________

____

Review of Systems

Head (*headache* [how often, quality, treatment outcome], *syncope, trauma*): ______________

____

Eyes (*vision problems, burning eyes, glasses, last eye exam, blocked tear duct, discharge, tearing, itching*): ______________

____

Ears (*difficulty hearing, discharge, earache, ringing or buzzing*): ______________________

____

Mouth and throat (*sore throat, lesions, toothache, caries, last dental visit*): ______________________

____

Respiratory system (*frequent colds, nosebleeds, cough, pneumonia, asthma, shortness of breath, sinusitis, hay fever*): ______

____

Cardiovascular system (*heart problems, hypertension, chest pain, cyanosis, shortness of breath, murmurs, edema*): ______

____

____

Gastrointestinal system (*nausea, vomiting, diarrhea, constipation, flatulence, abdominal pain, loss of appetite, weight loss or gain, rectal pain or bleeding*): ______________________________

____

Urinary tract (*dysuria, urinary frequency, urgency, nocturia, difficulty voiding, urinary retention, CVA pain*): __________

____

____

Reproductive system (*prostatitis, penile discharge* [color, character, amount], *lesions on penis, testicular self-exam, testicular pain, lumps, impotence, scrotal swelling, sexual activity, number of sexual partners, use of condoms, sexual satisfaction, history of STDs*): ______________________________

____

Musculoskeletal system (*joint pain, swelling, tremor, history of trauma, muscle weakness*): ______________

____

Integumentary system (*lesions* [describe character, locale, color], *changes in skin color, itching, hair loss, discoloration or pitting of nails, birthmarks, swollen glands*): ______________________________

____

Neurological system (*seizures, ataxia, tics, tremors, paralysis*): ______________________________

____

Hematopoietic system (*anemia, bleeding tendencies, bruise easily, transfusions* [when, why]): ______________

____

Immunologic system (*frequent infections, HIV infection, use of immunosuppressives*): ______________

____

Immunization status: ______________________________

____

Physical Examination

Height and weight: ______________________________

Vital signs (*T, P, R, B/P*): ______________________________

General appearance (*posture, gait, deformities, hygiene*): ______________________________

____

Skin (*include hair and nails*): ______________________________

____

Head and neck (*lymph nodes, face*): ______________________________

____

Eyes: ______________________________

Ears: ______________________________

Nose and sinuses: ______________________________

Mouth and throat (*lips, gums, palate, pharynx, tongue, teeth*): ______________________________

____

Chest:

Breast examination: ______

Heart: ______

Lungs: ______

Abdomen: ______

Genitalia (*including anus and rectum, prostate*): ______

Musculoskeletal system (*extremities, spine, joints, muscles*): ______

Nervous system (*cranial nerves, DTRs, temperature, kinesthetic sense*): ______

Results of screening and other tests: ______

Psychological Considerations

Self-image, level of self-esteem: ______

History of mental illness: ______

Emotional mood or state (*current and recent changes*): ______

Level of orientation: ______

Coping (*strategies used, effectiveness*): ______

Recent experience of significant loss (*death, divorce, relocation, effects*): ______

Suicide ideation: ______

Communication with others (*extent, adequacy*): ______

Interpersonal relationships (*extent, satisfaction*): ______

Stress (*sources, coping skills, support*): ______

Evidence of physical or emotional abuse: ______

Physical Environmental Considerations

Where does the client live? ______

Is there adequate space and privacy in the home? ______

Are safety hazards present in the home? ______ If so, what are they? ______

______

Are there safety hazards present in the work setting? ______ If so, what are they? ______

______

Are there pets in the home? (*What kind? How many? Inside or outside?*) ______

______

What is the neighborhood like? (*Describe safety, pollutants, etc.*) ______

______

Sociocultural Considerations

Education (*formal education, health knowledge, special learning needs*): ______

______

Income (*source, adequacy, budgeting skills*): ______

______

Social support network (*components, adequacy, use, marital status, character of marital relationship*): ______

______

Cultural practices influencing health: ______

______

Gender socialization and effects on health: ______

Family responsibilities and effects on health: ______

Extent of social support for healthy behavior: ______

______

Religious affiliation (*importance/influence on health*): ______

______

Adequacy of adult role models: ______

______

Employment (*current and past, hazards, job change pattern*): ______

______

Access to transportation: ______

Behavioral Considerations

Consumption Patterns

Usual diet (*meal pattern, preferences, preparation, nutritional adequacy, special needs, cultural restrictions*): ______

______

______

Use of alcohol, tobacco, other drugs: ______

______

Use of caffeine: ____

____

Use of medications (*type, appropriateness*): ____

____

Rest and Exercise

Sleep patterns: ____

____

Type and amount of exercise: ____

____

Leisure (*type of activity, hazards posed*): ____

____

Other

Sexual activity (*frequency, use of condoms, sexual orientation, multiple partners, sexual practices*): ______________________

____

Use of seat belts, other safety devices: ____

____

Health System Considerations

Use of primary prevention services (*general and dental*): ____

____

Attitudes toward health and health care: ____

____

Usual source of health care: ____

____

Health care financing (*type, adequacy*): ____

____

Barriers to care: ____

____

Use of health care services (*appropriateness*): ____

____

(For guidelines related to nursing diagnoses, planning, implementation, and evaluation of interventions for men use pages 35–36 of the *Family Health Assessment and Intervention Guide.*)

FUNCTIONAL HEALTH STATUS INVENTORY

Description: This inventory is intended to assist the community health nurse to assess clients' functional abilities. It addresses function in relation to basic, instrumental, and advanced activities of daily living.

Appropriate populations: Adult clients. May be particularly useful for home health clients and those with chronic or disabling conditions. May also be used to assess the functional status of clients with dementia or other mental and emotional health problems.

Data sources and data collection strategies: Data may be collected via interviews with clients or significant others or through observation of client abilities.

Use of information: Information gleaned from the inventory can be used to identify areas where nursing intervention is needed for clients to function more effectively. Data are also used to tailor nursing interventions for other health problems to clients' capabilities.

FUNCTIONAL HEALTH STATUS INVENTORY

Activity	Status	
Basic Activities of Daily Living	**Yes**	**No**
Feeding		
Can the client feed him- or herself?	❑	❑
Does the client have difficulty chewing?	❑	❑
Does the client have difficulty swallowing?	❑	❑
Bathing		
Can the client get into or out of the bathtub or shower?	❑	❑
Can the client manipulate soap and washcloth?	❑	❑
Can the client wash his or her hair without assistance?	❑	❑
Can the client effectively dry all body parts?	❑	❑
Dressing		
Can the client remember what articles of clothing should be put on first?	❑	❑
Can the client dress him- or herself?	❑	❑
Can the client bend and reach to put on shoes and stockings?	❑	❑
Can the client manipulate buttons and zippers?	❑	❑
Are modifications in clothing required to facilitate dressing (e.g., front opening dresses)?	❑	❑
Is arm and shoulder movement adequate to put on and remove sleeves?	❑	❑
Can the client comb his or her hair?	❑	❑
Can the client apply makeup if desired?	❑	❑
Toileting		
Is the client mobile enough to reach the bathroom?	❑	❑
Is there urgency that may lead to incontinence?	❑	❑
Can the client remove clothing in order to urinate or defecate?	❑	❑
Can the client position him- or herself on or in front of the toilet?	❑	❑
Can the client rise from a sitting position on the toilet?	❑	❑
Is the client able to clean him- or herself effectively after urinating or defecating?	❑	❑
Can the client replace clothing after urinating or defecating?	❑	❑
Transfer		
Is the client able to get from a lying to a sitting position unassisted?	❑	❑
Is the client able to stand from a sitting position without support or assistance?	❑	❑
Is the client able to sit or lie down without help?	❑	❑
Instrumental Activities of Daily Living		
Shopping		
Is the client able to transport him- or herself to shopping facilities?	❑	❑
Can the client navigate within a shopping facility?	❑	❑
Can the client lift products from shelves?	❑	❑
Can the client effectively handle money?	❑	❑
Can the client carry purchases from store to car and from car to home?	❑	❑
Is the client able to store purchases appropriately?	❑	❑
Laundry		
Can the client collect dirty clothes for washing?	❑	❑
Is the client able to sort clothes to be washed from those to be dry cleaned?	❑	❑
Can the client sort clothes by color?	❑	❑
Can the client access laundry facilities?	❑	❑
Can the client manipulate containers of soap, bleach, and so on?	❑	❑
Can the client lift wet clothing from washer to dryer or hang wet items to dry?	❑	❑

Activity	Status: Yes	Status: No
Is the client able to hang or fold clean clothes as needed?	❑	❑
Can the client put clean clothing in closets or drawers?	❑	❑
Cooking		
Is the client capable of planning well-balanced meals?	❑	❑
Can the client safely operate kitchen utensils and appliances (e.g., stove, can opener)?	❑	❑
Can the client reach dishes, pots, and pans needed for cooking and serving food?	❑	❑
Can the client clean vegetables and fruits, chop foods, etc.?	❑	❑
Is the client able to carry prepared foods to the table?	❑	❑
Housekeeping		
Can the client identify the need for housecleaning chores (e.g., when the tub needs to be cleaned)?	❑	❑
Is the client able to do light housekeeping (e.g., dusting, vacuuming, cleaning toilet)?	❑	❑
Is the client able to do heavy chores (e.g., scrub floors, wash windows)?	❑	❑
Is the client able to do yard maintenance, if needed?	❑	❑
Taking Medication		
Can the client remember to take medications as directed?	❑	❑
Is the client able to open medication bottles?	❑	❑
Can the client swallow oral medication, administer injections, and so on, as needed?	❑	❑
Managing Money		
Can the client effectively budget his or her income?	❑	❑
Is the client able to write checks?	❑	❑
Can the client balance a checking account?	❑	❑
Can the client remember to pay bills when due and record payment?	❑	❑
Advanced Activities of Daily Living		
Social Activity		
Does the client have a group of people with whom he or she can socialize?	❑	❑
Is the client able to transport him- or herself to social events?	❑	❑
Can the client see and hear well enough to interact socially with others?	❑	❑
Does the client tire too easily to engage in social activities?	❑	❑
Is social interaction impeded by fears of incontinence or embarrassment over financial difficulties?	❑	❑
Occupation		
Can the client carry out occupational responsibilities as needed?	❑	❑
Recreation		
Does the client have the physical strength and mobility to engage in desired recreational pursuits?	❑	❑
Does the client have the financial resources to engage in desired recreational pursuits?	❑	❑
Does the client have other people with whom to engage in recreation?	❑	❑
Does the client have access to recreational activities (e.g., transportation)?	❑	❑

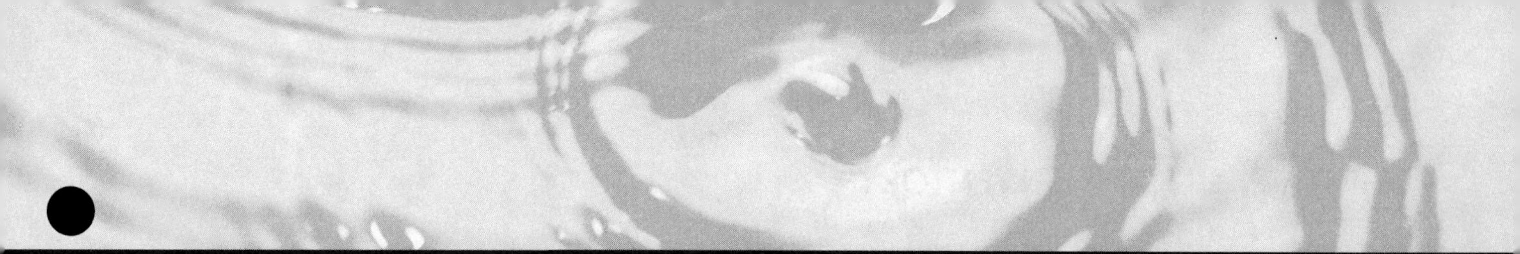

COGNITIVE FUNCTION INVENTORY

Description: This assessment guide is intended to assist the community health nurse to assess clients' cognitive function.

Appropriate populations: Adult clients who may be at risk for diminished cognitive function, particularly those who have evidence of dementia. May also be used with depressed clients or those with other mental or emotional illness. Assessment data should be interpreted within clients' cultural context.

Data sources and data collection strategies: Data may be collected via interviews with clients or significant others or through observation of client abilities.

Use of information: Information gleaned from the assessment is used to develop nursing interventions to improve clients' cognitive status when possible and to design nursing interventions for other health problems that are congruent with clients' cognitive abilities.

COGNITIVE FUNCTION INVENTORY

Assessment Area	Status	
	Yes	No
Attention Span		
Does the client focus on a single activity to completion?	❑	❑
Does the client move from activity to activity without completing any?	❑	❑
Concentration		
Is the client able to answer questions without wandering from the topic?	❑	❑
Does the client ignore irrelevant stimuli while focusing on a task?	❑	❑
Is the client easily distracted from a subject or task by external stimuli?	❑	❑
Intelligence		
Does the client understand directions and explanations given in everyday language?	❑	❑
Is the client able to perform basic mathematical calculations?	❑	❑
Judgment		
Does the client engage in action appropriate to the situation?	❑	❑
Are client behaviors based on an awareness of environmental conditions and possible consequences of action?	❑	❑
Are the client's plans and goals realistic?	❑	❑
Can the client effectively budget income?	❑	❑
Is the client safe driving a car?	❑	❑
Learning Ability		
Is the client able to retain instructions for a new activity?	❑	❑
Can the client recall information provided?	❑	❑
Is the client able to correctly demonstrate new skills?	❑	❑
Memory		
Is the client able to remember and describe recent events in some detail?	❑	❑
Is the client able to describe events from the past in some detail?	❑	❑
Orientation		
Can the client identify him- or herself by name?	❑	❑
Is the client aware of where he or she is?	❑	❑
Does the client recognize the identity and function of those around him or her?	❑	❑
Does the client know what day and time it is?	❑	❑
Is the client able to separate past, present, and future?	❑	❑
Perception		
Are the client's responses appropriate to the situation?	❑	❑
Does the client exhibit evidence of hallucinations or illusions?	❑	❑
Are explanations of events consistent with the events themselves?	❑	❑
Can the client reproduce simple figures?	❑	❑
Problem Solving		
Is the client able to recognize problems that need resolution?	❑	❑
Can the client envision alternative solutions to a given problem?	❑	❑
Can the client weigh alternative solutions and select one appropriate to the situation?	❑	❑
Can the client describe activities needed to implement the solution?	❑	❑
Psychomotor Ability		
Does the client exhibit repetitive movements that interfere with function?	❑	❑

Assessment Area	Status	
	Yes	No
Reaction Time		
Does the client take an unusually long time to respond to questions or perform motor activities?	❑	❑
Does the client respond to questions before the question is completed?	❑	❑
Social Intactness		
Are the client's interactions with others appropriate to the situation?	❑	❑
Is the client able to describe behaviors appropriate and inappropriate to a given situation?	❑	❑

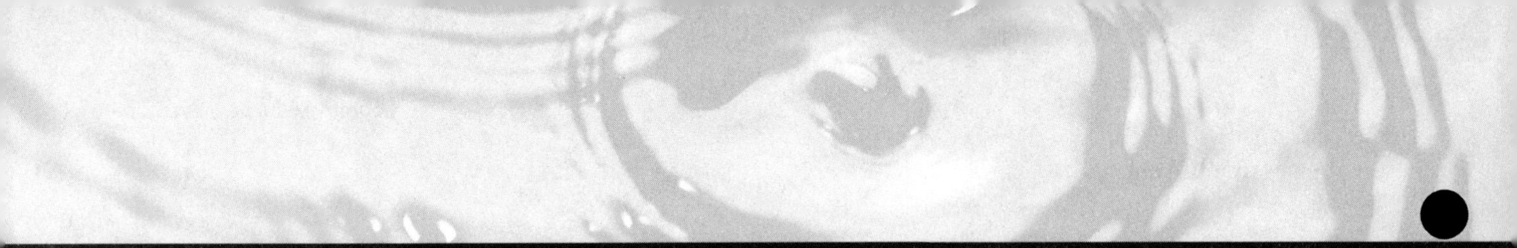

HOME SAFETY INVENTORY—OLDER ADULT

Description: This tool is designed to assist the community health nurse to identify safety hazards in the home of an older client.

Appropriate populations: The tool is designed specifically for use with older adults, but can be modified for use with other clients. For example, the inventory could be used to assess the safety of the home situation for a client with a disability, or to assess factors affecting the safety of groups of older persons. Many of the items are also relevant to home safety for all clients whatever their age or health status and can be used to identify general safety hazards present in the home or other settings.

Data sources and data collection strategies: Information on areas addressed by the *Home Safety Inventory* can be obtained by interviews with clients or other family members or by observation of the home setting.

Use of information: The results of the inventory can be used to educate individual clients or families regarding home safety issues and to motivate changes in environmental conditions to promote safety in the home. The inventories can also be completed by groups of people and the results used to initiate home safety education.

HOME SAFETY INVENTORY—OLDER ADULT

Safety Consideration	**Yes**	**No**
1. Lighting adequate on stairs?	☐	☐
2. Stair rails present and in good repair?	☐	☐
3. Nonskid surfaces on stairs?	☐	☐
4. Throw rugs present safety hazard?	☐	☐
5. Crowded living area presents safety hazard?	☐	☐
6. Tub rails installed?	☐	☐
7. Tub has nonskid surface?	☐	☐
8. Space heaters present safety hazard?	☐	☐
9. Adequate provision made for refrigeration of food?	☐	☐
10. Medications kept in appropriately labeled containers with readable print?	☐	☐
11. Toxic substances have labels with readable print and are stored well away from food?	☐	☐
12. Home is adequately ventilated and heated?	☐	☐
13. Neighborhood is safe?	☐	☐
14. Fire and police notified of older person in home?	☐	☐

HEALTH ASSESSMENT AND INTERVENTION GUIDE—OLDER ADULT

Description: This assessment guide is intended to assist the community health nurse to assess the health status of older clients. It is framed in terms of the nursing process and directs assessment, diagnosis, planning, implementation, and evaluation of community health nursing care for older adults. The assessment component of the tool reflects the six dimensions of health included in the dimensions model of community health nursing.

Appropriate populations: All older adult clients. May also be used with groups of older adults to identify problems common in population groups.

Data sources and data collection strategies: Interviews with or observations of older clients and physical examination may be used to obtain most of the assessment data included in the tool. For older clients who are cognitively impaired, information may be obtained in interviews with significant others. Medical and other records may also be a source of assessment data.

Use of information: The information gleaned from the assessment by the community health nurse is used to plan individualized nursing interventions to meet the health needs of the older adult client.

HEALTH ASSESSMENT AND INTERVENTION GUIDE—OLDER ADULT

Client's name: ______________________________ Phone: ______________

Address: ____

Assessment

Biophysical Considerations

Physiologic Function

Perceptions of personal health: ______________________________

____

Review of Systems (Include Effects of Aging)

Eyes (*visual impairment, use of glasses*): ______________________________

____

Ears (*hearing impairment, use of hearing aid*): ______________________________

____

Mouth and throat (*dentures* [fit, use], *dry mouth, bleeding gums*): ______________________________

____

Integumentary system (*skin integrity, fragility, dryness, itching, lesions, bruises, bleeding, skin color changes, hair distribution, thickened nails; hair, nail, and skin care practices; temperature of extremities, decreased perspiration*): ________

____

____

Respiratory system (*shortness of breath with exertion, cyanosis, emphysema, cough*): ______________________________

____

Cardiovascular system (*history of heart disease, palpitations, hypertension, effect of activity on heart rate, edema, fatigue, orthostatic hypotension, varicosities, venous stasis ulcers*): ______________________________

____

Gastrointestinal system (*flatulence, constipation, heartburn, rectal bleeding, incontinence, dysphagia, appetite, ability to chew*): ______________________________

____

Musculoskeletal system (*mobility, joint swelling, pain, use of cane or other device, history of fractures, kyphosis, scoliosis*):

____

____

____

Neurological system (*seizures, ataxia, tics, tremors, paralysis, diminished sense of smell, touch, heat sensation, taste, numbness or tingling*): ______________________________

____

____

Reproductive system (*decreased libido*): ______

- Male (*erectile dysfunction, prostatitis*): ______
- Female (*onset of menopause, menopausal symptoms, use of HRT, history of hysterectomy or breast cancer, last Pap smear, mammogram*): ______

Urinary system (*frequency, urgency, incontinence, color, odor, nocturia*): ______

Immunologic system (*frequent infection, HIV infection, use of immunosuppressives*): ______

Hematopoietic system (*anemia, epistaxis, bleeding tendencies*): ______

Existence of acute and chronic health problems (*diagnosis, status, treatment, effects*): ______

Functional abilities related to:

Bathing: ______

Dressing: ______

Toileting: ______

Mobility: ______

Eating: ______

Bowel and bladder function: ______

Communicating: ______

Immunization status (*tetanus, diphtheria, pneumonia, influenza*): ______

Psychological Considerations

Mental status/orientation: ______

Changes in self-image due to aging, retirement: ______________________________

Adjustment to retirement: ______________________________

Sources of stress: ______________________________

Coping abilities: ______________________________

History of mental illness: ______________________________

Provision for privacy: ______________________________

Loss of loved ones: ______________________________

Life satisfaction: ______________________________

Preparation for death: ______________________________

Evidence of depression: ______________________________

Evidence of abuse or neglect: ______________________________

Physical Environmental Considerations

Safety hazards in home (see *Home Safety Inventory—Older Adult, p. 88*): ______________________________

Presence of safety features in home: ______________________________

Availability of resources in neighborhood: ______________________________

Neighborhood safety: ______________________________

Driving: ______________________________

Home maintenance and repair: ______________________________

Pets: ______________________________

Adequacy of heating, lighting, ventilation: ______________________________

Sociocultural Considerations

Social interaction and support network: ____________________

____

Social attitudes to the elderly and effects on health: ____________________

Income (*source, adequacy, ability to budget*): ____________________

____

Relationships with family: ____________________

____

Family responsibilities and effects on health: ____________________

____

Education level: ____________________

____

Religion and importance in client's life: ____________________

____

Culture and ethnicity and influence on client's health: ____________________

____

Possibility of institutionalization and client response: ____________________

____

Current employment and potential health effects: ____________________

____

Previous occupation and effects on health: ____________________

____

Access to transportation: ____________________

Access to goods and services (e.g., grocery stores): ____________________

____

Behavioral Considerations

Consumption Patterns

Nutrition (*adequacy for needs, special needs, appetite, meal pattern, food preferences and modes of preparation, food supplements, food storage, shopping practices*): ____________________

____

Use of tobacco, alcohol, or other drugs: ____________________

____

Use of medications (*type, appropriateness, effectiveness*): ____________________

____

Rest and Exercise

Sleep patterns: ____________________

____

Exercise: ______________________________

____

Leisure Activities

Preferred leisure pursuits: ______________________________

____

Opportunity for leisure activities: ______________________________

____

Sexuality

Opportunity for intimacy: ______________________________

____

Alternative modes of meeting sexual needs: ______________________________

____

Independence

Ability to care for self: ______________________________

____

Ability to make independent decisions: ______________________________

____

Other safety practices: ______________________________

Other health-related practices (e.g., mammogram, prostate exam): ______________________________

Driving practices/safety: ______________________________

Health System Considerations

Source of health care: ______________________________

____

Health care financing (*Medicare, insurance*): ______________________________

____

Financing of prescription medications: ______________________________

Use of health care services: ______________________________

____

Barriers to obtaining health care: ______________________________

____

(For guidelines related to nursing diagnoses, planning, implementation, and evaluation of interventions for older adults use pages 35–36 of the *Family Health Assessment and Intervention Guide*.)

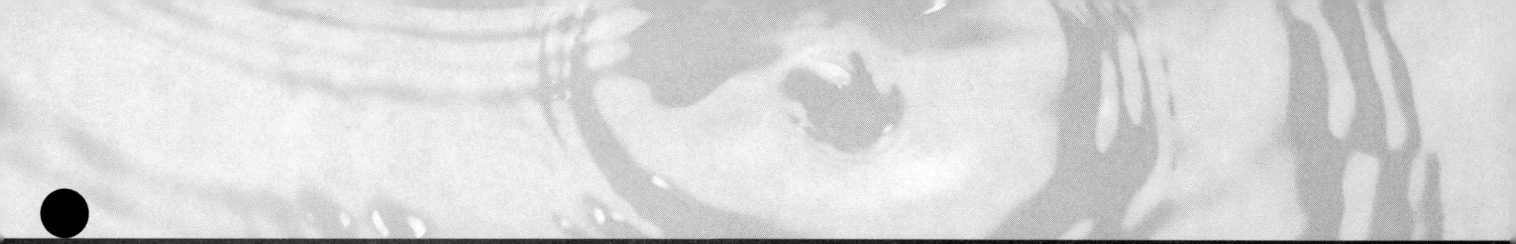

COMMUNITY HOUSING ASSESSMENT

Description: This tool is designed for use in assessing the availability and affordability of housing in the community.

Appropriate populations: Local population groups, communities, or neighborhoods.

Data sources and data collection strategies: Census data and information collected by local government agencies (e.g., housing authority, chamber of commerce, etc.) may be used to answer questions included in the tool.

Use of information: Information obtained through use of the assessment tool can be used to identify local housing issues and as a basis for planning to meet housing needs.

COMMUNITY HOUSING ASSESSMENT

What is the total number of housing units in the community? _______

What percentage is rental units? _______What percentage is owner occupied? _______

What is the typical percentage of housing units vacant at any point in time? _______

What is the total number of households in the population? _______

What is the average number of persons per household? _______

Is the number of housing units adequate to accommodate the number of people? _______

What is the median monthly cost of housing in the area? _______

What is the median income per household? _______

Is there a significant discrepancy between housing costs and median income? _______

What is the percentage of households with incomes below poverty level? _______

What percentage of households with incomes below 50% of poverty level spend 50% or more of their income on housing? _______

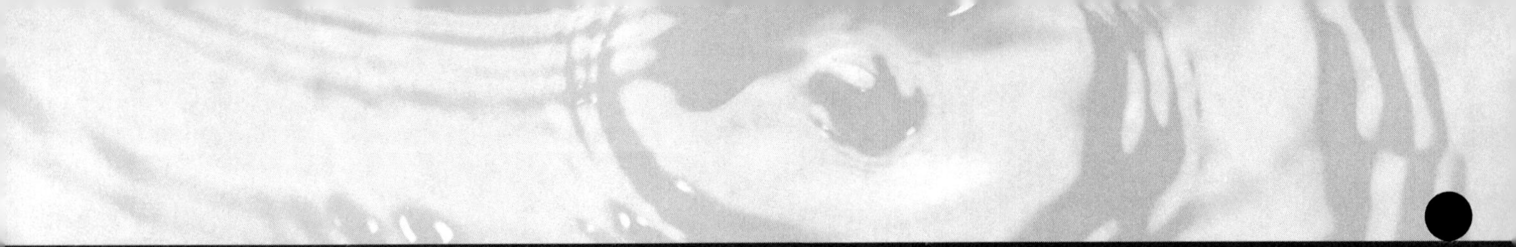

HOME HEALTH NURSING ASSESSMENT

Description: This tool can be used to assess the health needs of a client in a home health nursing situation. It is based on the dimensions model and assists the community health nurse to identify health problems in each of the six dimensions of health.

Appropriate populations: In any home visiting situation, but probably most useful with clients being followed for existing health problems, particularly chronic diseases.

Data sources and collection strategies: Data for the biophysical dimension segment of the tool are derived from observation, client interview, and elements of physical examination. Psychological, sociocultural, behavioral, and health system dimensions data are usually obtained during client interviews or observations. Data related to the physical environmental dimension are primarily obtained by observation of the home environment. Some data in each of the dimensions may be available from the referral source.

Use of information: Information collected can be used to identify client health needs and to plan appropriate interventions to be implemented during the home visit.

HOME HEALTH NURSING ASSESSMENT

Patient name: ____________________ Birth date: ____________________ Record #: ____________________

Address: ____

Phone number: ____

Biophysical Considerations

Male _______ Female _______

Primary medical diagnosis: ____

Past medical history: ____

____

____

____

General appearance: ____

____

Vital signs: Temp ___________ Pulse: Apical ________ Radial: _____ Respirations: _______

Weight: _________ Height: _______

Blood pressure: (1) Right arm—Supine _______ Sitting _______ Standing _______

(2) Left arm—Supine _______ Sitting _______ Standing _______

Hearing: Normal _______ Hearing impaired: _______ Deaf: _______

Uses hearing aid: R _______ L _______

Vision: Normal _______ Blind: _______ Limited _______

Uses glasses: Sometimes _______ Always _______

Developmental level: ____

Allergies:____

Functional abilities:

No problems: _______

Difficulty with: Bathing: _________ Dressing: __________ Toileting: _________

Mobility/transfer: __________ Eating: _________ Bowel control: _________ Bladder control: _________

Communication: __________ Meal preparation: __________ Housekeeping: ______ Shopping: _______

Use of assistive devices:____

Describe any limitations noted:____

Immunization status:____

Review of Systems/Physical Examination

Neurological: No problems _______ Oriented x _______ Headache _______ Vertigo_______Tremors _______

Seizures ________ Syncope ________ Paresthesias ________ Weakness________

LOC (describe):____

Cardiovascular: No problems ______ Palpitations ______ Fainting ______ Dizziness _______ Edema ______

Cyanosis ______ Neck vein distention _______ Chest pain _______ Pulse irregularity _______ Syncope ______

Circumoral pallor _______

Respiratory: No problems _______ Dyspnea _______ SOB _______ SOBOE _______ Orthopnea ________

Cough ________ Cyanosis ________ Pain ________ Sputum ________ IPPB ________ O_2 ________

Lung sounds (describe): ____

Gastrointestinal: No problems ______ Nausea _______ Vomiting _______ Anorexia _______ Bleeding _______

Pain _______ Diarrhea _______ Constipation ______ Incontinent _______ Distention _______ Aphagia _______

NGT _______ GT _______ JT _______ Bowel sounds (describe): ______________________________

Genitourinary: No problems _______ Frequency _______ Urgency _______ Pain _______ Burning _______

Nocturia _______ Hematuria _______ Difficulty urinating _______ Incontinent _______ Retention _______

Catheter _______

Integumentary: No problems _______ Cool _______ Warm _______ Diaphoresis _______ Pallor _______

Cyanosis_______ Flushing _______ Mottling _______ Jaundice _______ Pruritus _______ Petechiae _______

Dry _______ Decubitus _______ Pressure areas _______ Wound/incision (describe): ________________

Rash (describe): ______________________________ Bruises (describe): ___________________________

Turgor (describe): ____

Musculoskeletal: No problems _______ Joint swelling _______ Decreased ROM _______ Back pain _______

Reproductive: No problems ______ Impotence _______ Prostatitis _______ Discharge _______ Breast mass _______

Testicular mass _______ Decreased libido _______ Dysmenorrhea _______ Dyspareunia _______

Last Pap smear: _____________

Hematopoietic: No problems _______ Anemia _______ Epistaxis _______ Bruising _______

Venous access: Good _______ Fair _______ Poor _______

Immunologic: Frequent infection _______ Diminished immune status _______ HIV infection _______

Immunizations:____

Pain: None _______ Description ______________________________________

Intensity: 1+ (mild) _______ 2+ (discomfort) _______ 3+ (distressing) _______ 4+ (severe) _______

5+ (excruciating) _______

Analgesics taken _____________________ Dose _____________________ Frequency ______________

Effectiveness: ____

Degree of limitation due to pain: ______________________________________

Psychological Considerations

Mood: No problems _______ Depressed _______ Anxious _______ Restless _______ Uncooperative _______

Mentation: Alert _______ Confused _______ Disoriented _______

Coping: Adequate _______ Minimal _______ Inadequate _______

History of mental illness: ___________________________ Recent loss: ____________________

Life satisfaction: ____

History of family violence: ______________________________________

Sources of stress: ____

Physical Environmental Considerations

Type of residence: House _______ Apartment _______ Institution _______ Shelter _______ None _______

Ease of access: Stairs to climb _______ Ramp _______

Space: Adequate _______ Inadequate: _______

Distance to bathroom: ______________________________

Home safety: Adequate _______ Safety hazards present: ______________________________

Safety features in home: Childproof latches _________ Tub rail _________ Grounded outlets _________

Stair lights _________ Stair rails _________ Smoke alarm _________

Infection control hazards: ______________________________

Inadequate: Lighting _______ Heat _______ Ventilation _______ Air conditioning _______ Refrigeration _______

Cooking facilities _______ Plumbing _______ Waste disposal _______ Electricity _______

Use of space heaters: ______________________________

Storage of hazardous materials: ______________________________

Firearms in home: ______________________________

Home maintenance/repair: Adequate ________ Inadequate ________ Problems noted: ________________

Pets: Type ______________________________ Indoor _______ Outdoor _______

Neighborhood safety: ______________________________

Environmental pollutants: ______________________________

Sociocultural Considerations

Educational level: ______________________________ Income: ______________________________

Primary language: ______________________________ Interpreter: ______________________________

Religious affiliation: ______________________________ Ethnicity: ______________________________

Employed ________ Unemployed ________ Retired ________ Occupation(s): ______________________________

Single _______ Married _______ Divorced _______ Widowed _______

Other persons in home (*include ages, health problems, etc.*):

Quality of family interactions:

Opportunity for social interaction:

Social support network:

Cultural influences:

Availability of transportation:

Behavioral Considerations

Diet: Inadequate in: Calories _______ Protein _______ Iron _______ Potassium _______ Calcium _______

Vitamin A _______ Vitamin B complex _______ C _______ D _______ K _______ Fluid _______ Fiber _______

Excessive Fat _______ Calories _______ Sodium _______

Method of preparation: ______________________________

Typical meal pattern: ______________________________

Other substances: Alcohol use ______ Amount ______________________________

Illicit drug use ______ Type ______ Amount ______ Route ______________________________

Tobacco use ______ Type ______ Amount ______ Length of use ______________________________

Medications (include prescription and over-the-counter medications):

Medication	Dose	Frequency	Route	Purpose	Length of use
1.					
2.					
3.					
4.					
5.					

Sleep patterns:

Exercise:

Leisure activities:

Sexually active ______ Orientation: ______________ Satisfaction: ______________

Unsafe sexual practices: ______________________________

Other behaviors: Seat belt use ______ Contraceptive use ______________________________

Use of other safety equipment ______________________________

Health System Considerations

Usual source of health care: ______________________________

Source of health care funding: ______________________________

Use of preventive services: ______________________________

Attitudes toward health and health care: ______________________________

Barriers to access: ______________________________

HEALTH ASSESSMENT IN THE SCHOOL SETTING

Description: This tool is designed to assist the community health nurse to apply the dimensions model to the care of groups of clients in the school setting. It is intended to assess the health status of school populations rather than individual students or school personnel. Assistance in directing care of individuals in the school setting can be found in other assessment tools included in this book. (See the *Child and Adolescent Health Assessment and Intervention Guide* [pp. 52–58], *Health Assessment and Intervention Guide—Adult Woman* [pp. 65–70], *Health Assessment and Intervention Guide—Adult Man* [pp. 76–81], or *Health Assessment and Intervention Guide—Older Adult* [pp. 89–94].)

Appropriate populations: May be used with any school population from the preschool or day care setting to college. It can also be used with different cultural groups within school settings.

Data sources and data collection strategies: Sources of data used in the assessment of school health status will include reviews of school records; interviews with school personnel, parents, and students; interviews with representatives of other community agencies and organizations that interact with the school; and personal observations by the nurse. Surveys of students, staff, families, and community members may also be used to obtain information on health in the school setting.

Use of information: Information gleaned from the assessment of the health status of the school population will be used for a variety of purposes. One major use of the data is in the design of school health programs to meet identified health needs. Information may also be used to plan a health education curriculum in areas that address identified needs. Finally, information on the health status of school populations may be used to direct community planning efforts designed to improve the health status of the broader community or to enhance the effectiveness of school–community interaction with respect to health.

HEALTH ASSESSMENT IN THE SCHOOL SETTING

Assessment

Biophysical Considerations

Age, gender, and racial/ethnic composition of the school population: ______________________

Extent and severity of developmental delays among students: ______________________

Specific developmental considerations: ______________________

Presence of handicapping conditions: ______________________

Incidence of communicable disease *(students and staff)*: ______________________

Incidence and prevalence of chronic disease *(students and staff)*: ______________________

Prevalence of genetic predisposition to disease: ______________________

Immunization levels: ______________________

Psychological Considerations

Extent of connectedness to the school exhibited by students: ______________________

Organization of the school day (*appropriateness to needs, effects on health*): ______________________

Aesthetic quality of environment: ______________________

Relationships among students (*quality, appropriateness of adult monitoring*): ______________________

Prevalence of bullying or victimization in school population: ______________________

Teacher–student relations (*quality, extent*): ______________________

Teacher–teacher relations: ______________________

Discipline (*type, extent, appropriateness, consistency, fairness*): ______________________

Grading practices (*consistency, fairness*): ______________________

Parent–school relations (*quality, extent*): ____________________

____

Sources of stress in the school environment: ____________________

____

Prevalence of mental illness in the school population: ____________________

Physical Environmental Considerations

Traffic patterns around the school: ____________________

____

Exposure to school bus emissions: ____________________

Presence of safety belts in school buses: ____________________

Safety hazards in the neighborhood: ____________________

____

Use of pesticides and other poisons in the neighborhood: ____________________

____

Pollutants in the area of the school: ____________________

____

Fire or safety hazards in the school environment: ____________________

____

Use of toxic chemicals in labs, art classes, cleaning and maintenance: ____________________

____

Use of hazardous equipment in home economics or "shop" classes: ____________________

____

Broken glass in recreational areas: ____________________

____

Play equipment in poor repair: ____________________

____

Hard surfaces below play equipment: ____________________

____

Animals in the school environment: ____________________

____

Plant allergens or poisons in the school environment: ____________________

____

Adequacy of heating, lighting, cooling: ____________________

____

Noise levels: ____________________

____

Food sanitation practices: ______________________________

Toilet facilities (*adequacy, state of repair*): ______________________________

Cleaning of shower facilities: ______________________________

Isolation facilities for students with communicable diseases: ______________________________

Facilities and access for handicapped students or staff: ______________________________

Disaster potential in the environment around the school: ______________________________

Sociocultural Considerations

Community attitudes toward education and toward school: ______________________________

Community support of school program: ______________________________

Crime in neighborhood (*extent, effect on school and student health*): ______________________________

Funding (*source, extent, adequacy, priorities*): ______________________________

Home environment of students: ______________________________

Availability of before- and after-school care: ______________________________

Socioeconomic status of students, staff: ______________________________

Presence of intergroup conflicts: ______________________________

Prevalence of violence in the school environment: ______________________________

School policies related to violence: ______________________________

Potential for Internet exploitation of students: ______________________________

Ethnic/cultural background of staff, students: ______________________________

Education level of families and extent of health knowledge: ______________________________

Extent of homelessness among students: ____________________

____

Extent of parental involvement with the school: ____________________

Behavioral Considerations

Consumption Patterns

Quality of school meal programs: ____________________

____

Student/staff nutritional levels: ____________________

____

Special nutritional needs (*students or staff*): ____________________

____

Prevalence of food allergies in school population: ____________________

Nutrition knowledge (*extent among students, staff, parents*): ____________________

____

Extent of alcohol or drug use by students, staff, family members: ____________________

____

Extent of tobacco use by students, staff, family members: ____________________

____

School policies related to tobacco, drug, and alcohol use: ____________________

____

Medication use *(types, storage, dispensing policies)*: ____________________

____

Exercise and Leisure Activities

Rest and exercise patterns of school population: ____________________

____

Recreational opportunities (*type, age-appropriateness*): ____________________

____

Use of appropriate safety equipment: ____________________

____

Other

Sexual activity by students (*extent, use of contraceptives, use of condoms and other barrier devices*): ____________________

____

Use of safety devices (*seat belts*): ____________________

____

Prevalence of gambling in school population: ____________________

Prevalence of piercing/tattoos in the school population: ____________________

Health System Considerations

Health care services offered by school: ______________________________

____

Extent of use of school nurse and other school health services: ______________________________

____

Availability of community health care services (*physical and mental health*): ______________________________

____

Use of health care services by school population: ______________________________

____

Financing of health care services *(source, adequacy)*: ______________________________

____

Emphasis placed on health in school curriculum: ______________________________

____

Support of school health program by health care professionals in the community: ______________________________

____

Extent of coordination between school and community health services: ______________________________

____

School and community attitudes toward health and health care: ______________________________

____

(For guidelines related to nursing diagnoses, planning, implementation, and evaluation of interventions for school populations use pages 47–49 of the *Population Health Assessment and Intervention Guide.*)

WORK FITNESS INVENTORY

Description: This inventory is intended for use in determining the individual employee's fitness for a specific job. The inventory incorporates elements of the biophysical, psychological, physical environmental, sociocultural, behavioral, and health system dimensions of the dimensions model to assist health care providers in the occupational health setting to determine whether a given employee has the physical and mental capacity to perform certain tasks without endangering his or her health or the health and safety of others.

Appropriate populations: For use with individual employees.

Data sources and data collection strategies: Data may be obtained from interviews with employees and supervisors, specific tests of functional ability, laboratory test results, and review of the employee's job description. Additional data may be available from employee health records or from the records of other health care providers (with employee consent).

Use of information: Information derived from the inventory may be used to determine the appropriateness of initial hiring and placement decisions or an employee's fitness to return to work after an illness or injury. Information may also be used to help supervisors redesign an employee's position to prevent adverse health consequences. When information indicates a poor fit between the job and the employee, the nurse may also use this information to help the employee decide on career options that are more in keeping with his or her health status and capabilities.

WORK FITNESS INVENTORY

	Status: Yes	Status: No
Biophysical Considerations		
Does the employee have the physical stamina required for the job?	❑	❑
Does the employee have any mobility limitations that would interfere with performance?	❑	❑
Does the employee have sufficient joint mobility to do the job?	❑	❑
Does the employee have any postural limitations that would interfere with performance?	❑	❑
Does the employee have the required strength for the job?	❑	❑
Does the employee have the level of coordination required?	❑	❑
Does the employee have problems with balance that would interfere with performance?	❑	❑
Does the employee have any cardiorespiratory limitations?	❑	❑
Is there a possibility for unconsciousness that would create a safety hazard?	❑	❑
Does the employee have the required level of visual and auditory acuity?	❑	❑
Does the employee have communication and speech capabilities required by the job?	❑	❑
Will the employee's age put him or her at increased risk of injury or illness?	❑	❑
Does the job involve shift work that will adversely affect biological rhythms?	❑	❑
Psychological Considerations		
Does the employee have the requisite level of cognitive function (e.g., memory, critical thinking)?	❑	❑
Will the employee's mental or emotional state (e.g., depression) interfere with performance?	❑	❑
Does the employee have the required motivational level?	❑	❑
Does the job involve high levels of stress?	❑	❑
Does the employee have effective stress management skills?	❑	❑
Does the employee have little control over his or her work?	❑	❑
Is there any possibility that the employee might endanger self or others?	❑	❑
Physical Environmental Considerations		
Does the employee require assistive aids or appliances? Will work processes or setting need to be adapted to accommodate these aids (e.g., space for a wheelchair)?	❑	❑
Are there risk factors in the work setting that would adversely affect the employee?	❑	❑
Does the job involve extreme weather exposures that would adversely affect the employee?	❑	❑
If the employee is pregnant or of childbearing age, are there reproductive risks present in the work setting or job activities?	❑	❑
Does the work setting pose problems for emergency evacuation of a disabled employee?	❑	❑
Sociocultural Considerations		
Will the employee be working alone?	❑	❑
Will working alone have detrimental effects on the employee's physical or mental health?	❑	❑
Is the employee likely to be subjected to discrimination or sexual harassment?	❑	❑
Does the employee have the interpersonal skills required?	❑	❑
Does the job involve travel? Will travel adversely affect the employee's health?	❑	❑
Will travel or job schedule (e.g., shift work) conflict with family responsibilities?	❑	❑
Behavioral Considerations		
Does the employee have special dietary needs that cannot be met in the work setting?	❑	❑
Does the employee have a substance abuse problem that would interfere with performance?	❑	❑
Does the employee have a substance abuse problem that would pose a safety hazard to self or others?	❑	❑
Does the employee engage in behaviors (e.g., smoking) that will interact negatively with other exposures in the work setting?	❑	❑
Does the job promote the necessary level of physical activity to maintain health?	❑	❑
Does the job involve strenuous physical activity beyond the employee's capability?	❑	❑
Does the employee have specific manual skills required for the job?	❑	❑

	Status	
	Yes	No
Health System Considerations		
Are there treatment effects that will interfere with performance (e.g., drowsiness due to medications)?	❑	❑
Will treatment plans interfere with performance (e.g., nausea due to chemotherapy)?	❑	❑
What is the employee's prognosis? Will existing conditions improve or deteriorate?	❑	❑
Does the employee have any special health needs to be met in the work setting?	❑	❑

HEALTH ASSESSMENT IN THE WORK SETTING

Description: This tool is intended to assist community health nurses working in occupational health settings to identify health problems present in employee populations. The tool also facilitates planning, implementation, and evaluation of nursing interventions for this population.

Appropriate populations: Groups of employees in business and industrial settings. May be applied to both manufacturing and service employment settings and with small or large groups of employees. Assessment of the health status of individual employees is better conducted using the *Health Assessment and Intervention Guide—Adult Woman* [pp. 65–70], *Health Assessment and Intervention Guide—Adult Man* [pp. 76–81], or *Health Assessment and Intervention Guide—Older Adult* [pp. 89–94].

Data sources and data collection strategies: Data for assessing health needs in the occupational setting may be obtained from a variety of sources including company safety and injury records, employment compensation and insurance claims, employee health records, and interviews with employees and management personnel. Results of routine screening of employees also provide health status information. Health care providers in the community who provide services to employees may be another source of information. Additional information may be obtained through personal observation of working conditions, use of safety precautions, and so on. Because of the magnitude and complexity of the assessment data needed, the community health nurse may be one of several people collecting data. Community health nurses, however, are ideally suited to initiate and coordinate data collection as well as to guide the interpretation and use of the data obtained.

Use of information: Information on employee health status is used to derive community nursing diagnoses that direct the planning, implementation, and evaluation of health programs in the work setting. Information may also be used to identify larger community health concerns and to initiate efforts to address those concerns.

HEALTH ASSESSMENT IN THE WORK SETTING

Assessment

Biophysical Considerations

Age, gender, and racial/ethnic composition of the employee population: ______________________

____

Prevalence of disability in the employee population: ______________________

____

Injury incidence, type, and long-term effects in the employee population: ______________________

____

Incidence and prevalence of disease *(occupational, communicable, and chronic)*: ______________________

____

Prevalence of genetic predisposition to disease: ______________________

____

Extent of absenteeism: ______________________

____

Number and type of workers' compensation claims: ______________________

____

Immunization levels *(diphtheria, pertussis, tetanus, varicella, measles, rubella [especially for women of childbearing age], influenza, pneumonia)*: ______________________

____

Results of periodic screening tests: ______________________

____

Psychological Considerations

Organization of the workday (*shift work, breaks, overtime*): ______________________

____

Aesthetic quality of environment: ______________________

____

Relationships among employees: ______________________

____

Relationships between employees and management: ______________________

____

Employee morale: ______________________

____

Supervisor leadership styles (*appropriateness*): ______________________

____

Employee evaluation practices (*consistency, fairness*): ______

Job satisfaction: ______

Extent of employee control of job: ______

Extent of emotional labor by workforce: ______

Extent and sources of stress in the workplace (*sources, coping abilities*): ______

Extent of work/home role conflict: ______

Availability of stress management programs: ______

Prevalence of emotional problems/mental illness in the employee population: ______

Availability of employee assistance programs: ______

Physical Environmental Considerations

Typical commute (*distance, traffic*): ______

Safety of parking areas: ______

Use of pesticides and other poisons in the work environment: ______

Pollutants in the work environment: ______

Fire or safety hazards: ______

Potential for toxic substance exposures: ______

Use of hazardous equipment: ______

Extent of exposure to extreme weather conditions: ______

Potential for falls: ______

Need for heavy lifting: ______

Extent of repetitive motion in work: ____________________

Ergonomics of workstations: ____________________

____

Animals/insects in the work environment: ____________________

____

Plant allergens or poisons in the work environment: ____________________

____

Company policies to minimize safety hazards (*presence, enforcement, efficacy*): ____________________

____

Adequacy of heating, lighting, cooling, ventilation: ____________________

____

Noise levels: ____________________

____

Sanitation of food preparation and storage areas: ____________________

____

Toilet facilities (*adequacy, state of repair*): ____________________

____

Availability of shower facilities for dealing with external toxic substance exposures: ____________________

____

Facilities and access for handicapped employees: ____________________

____

Potential for disaster: ____________________

____

Sociocultural Considerations

Economic stability of employing organization: ____________________

____

Salary levels (*adequacy, equity*): ____________________

____

Health benefits available: ____________________

____

Community attitudes toward employing organization: ____________________

____

Crime in neighborhood: ____________________

____

Potential for violence in the work setting: ____________________

____

Occupational effects on family responsibilities: ____________________

____

Childcare availability: ____________________

Family leave policies: ____________________

Intergroup conflicts/discrimination: ____________________

Cultural background of employees and effects on health: ____________________

Languages spoken by employees: ____________________

Education level of employees and extent of health knowledge: ____________________

Extent of coworker support/cohesion ____________________

Coworker support for healthy behaviors: ____________________

Management support for healthy behaviors: ____________________

Applicability/enforcement of OSHA standards: ____________________

Applicability/enforcement of industry-specific standards: ____________________

Applicability/enforcement of ADA standards: ____________________

Implementation of health-related policies: ____________________

Extent of sexual harassment: ____________________

Behavioral Considerations

Consumption Patterns

Nutritional quality of food services: ____________________

Employee nutrition levels: ____________________

Special nutrition needs: ____________________

Nutrition knowledge: ____________________

Extent of alcohol or drug use by employees: ______________________________

____

Tobacco use *(extent, policies, cessation programs)*: ______________________________

____

Medication use by employees: ______________________________

____

Leisure Activities

Rest and activity patterns of employees: ______________________________

____

Opportunity for physical activity: ______________________________

____

Other

Types of work performed and health effects: ______________________________

____

Adequacy of safety policies and procedures: ______________________________

____

Use of appropriate safety equipment and procedures: ______________________________

____

Extent of sickness presenteeism in the employee population: ______________________________

Health System Considerations

Health care services offered in work setting: ______________________________

____

Availability of other health care services: ______________________________

____

Use of health care services by employee population: ______________________________

____

Funding of health care services *(adequacy, source)*: ______________________________

____

Extent of employee health insurance coverage: ______________________________

Employee attitudes toward health and health services: ______________________________

____

Availability of health promotion programs and type: ______________________________

____

Degree of emphasis placed on health promotion/illness prevention in the work setting: ______________________________

____

Adequacy of procedures to control and monitor toxic exposures: ______________________________

____

Adequacy of surveillance systems to detect hazardous exposures/adverse health effects: ______________________________

____

Extent of coordination between internal and external health care systems: ______________________________

____

(For guidelines related to nursing diagnoses, planning, implementation, and evaluation of interventions for employee populations use pages 47–49 of the *Population Health Assessment and Intervention Guide.*)

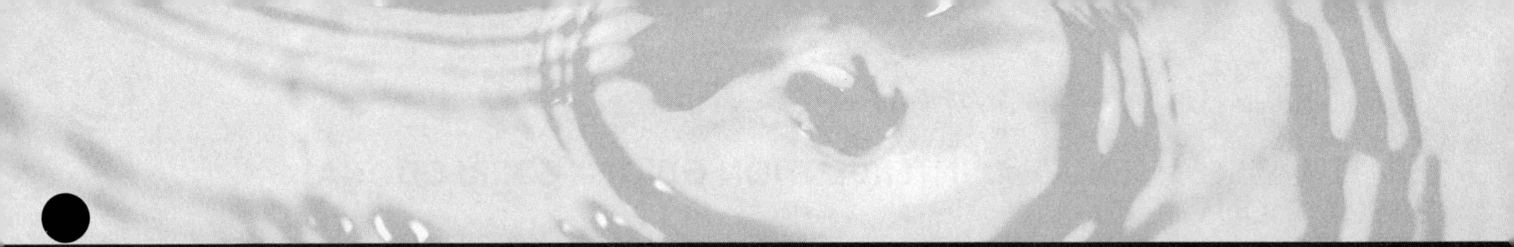

HEALTH ASSESSMENT AND INTERVENTION GUIDE—CORRECTIONAL POPULATIONS

Description: This assessment guide is intended to assist the community health nurse to assess the health needs of correctional populations, including both inmates and corrections personnel, and to direct the planning, implementation, and evaluation of nursing interventions to meet identified population health needs. The assessment component of the tool is based on the six dimensions of health in the dimensions model of community health nursing.

Appropriate populations: For assessment of population groups rather than individual clients in a corrections setting. Assessment tools provided elsewhere in this book (see *Child and Adolescent Health Assessment and Intervention Guide* [pp. 52–58], *Health Assessment and Intervention Guide—Adult Woman* [pp. 65–70], *Health Assessment and Intervention Guide—Adult Man* [pp. 76–81], or *Health Assessment and Intervention Guide—Older Adult* [pp. 89–94]) may be used to assess specific individuals within the population.

Data sources and data collection strategies: Information required to assess the correctional population may be obtained from facility records, review of individual client records, observation, and interviews with inmates and staff.

Use of information: The information gleaned from the assessment is used by the community health nurse to make nursing diagnoses and to plan, implement, and evaluate nursing care to address the health needs of the correctional population.

HEALTH ASSESSMENT AND INTERVENTION GUIDE—CORRECTIONAL POPULATIONS

Assessment

Biophysical Considerations

Age and Gender Composition of the Population

Gender	<19 years	19–29 years	30–59 years	60–69 years	70–79 years	80+ years
Male						
Female						

Ethnic Composition of the Population

Ethnicity	Percentage
African American	
Asian	
Caucasian	
Hispanic	
Native American	
Other	

What communicable diseases are prevalent among inmates/staff? ____________________

____

What chronic health problems are prevalent among inmates/staff? ____________________

____

What is the prevalence of disability among inmates/staff? ____________________

What is the prevalence of pregnancy among inmates/staff? ____________________

How adequate are immunization levels among inmates/staff? ____________________

Psychological Considerations

What procedures are in place for dealing with suicidal ideation or attempts? ____________________

____

Are these procedures followed? ____________________

What is the incidence of suicide attempts in the inmate population? ____________________

What is the prevalence of depression in the population? ____________________

What is the incidence rate for sexual assault among inmates? ____________________

Are there inmates in the setting under sentence of death? ____________________

Are there terminally ill inmates in the population? ____________________

What is the prevalence of mental illness among inmates/staff? ____________________

Physical Environmental Considerations

What health or safety hazards are present in the correctional facility? ____________________________________

____

Is there potential for disaster in the area? _______ If so, what types of disasters might be anticipated?____________

____

Is there a disaster plan? _______ How adequate is the plan for addressing potential disasters?_______________

____

____

Sociocultural Considerations

What are the attitudes of health and correctional personnel toward inmates? ______________________________

____

What is the attitude of the surrounding community toward the facility? Toward inmates? ____________________

____

What family concerns influence the health of inmates/staff? ____

____

Are there intergroup conflicts within the population? ____

What is the prevalence of violence in the setting? ____

What factors in the setting contribute to violence? ____

____

How transient is the inmate population? ____

Are inmates employed in the correctional setting? _______ Are they employed outside the setting? _______ What types of work are done? ____

What health hazards, if any, are posed by the type of work done? ____________________________________

____

How do security concerns affect the ability of health care personnel to provide services? ____________________

____

Behavioral Considerations

Are there inmates with special nutritional needs? _______ What are their needs? _________________________

____

How well are nutritional needs being met? ____

____

What is the nutritional quality of food served in the correctional setting? _______________________________

____

What are the health-related behaviors of the correctional population? How do they affect health? _____________

____

____

How are medications dispensed in the correctional setting? ______________________________

____

What procedures are used to prevent inmates from selling medications or accumulating them for use in suicide attempts? ______________________________

What is the prevalence of unsafe sexual activity in the correctional setting? ______________________________

____

What is the availability of condoms in the correctional setting? ______________________________

____

To what extent are appropriate safety practices and equipment used by the correctional population?____________

____

Health System Considerations

What health services are offered in the correctional setting? ______________________________

____

____

Are internal health services adequate to meet identified health needs? _______ If not, what additional services are needed? ______________________________

What isolation procedures are used to prevent the spread of communicable diseases? ______________________________

____

Is health care funding adequate to meet health needs? ______________________________

Are inmates charged a fee for health care services? _______ If yes, how does this affect access to health care?_______

____

What is the quality of interaction between internal and external health care services?______________________________

____

How adequate is the emergency response capability of the correctional facility (e.g., to myocardial infarction, stab wound, disaster event)? ______________________________

____

What procedures are in place to communicate inmates' health needs and plans of care to other agencies upon transfer or release? ______________________________

____

(For guidelines related to nursing diagnoses, planning, implementation, and evaluation of interventions for correctional populations use pages 47–49 of the *Population Health Assessment and Intervention Guide.*)

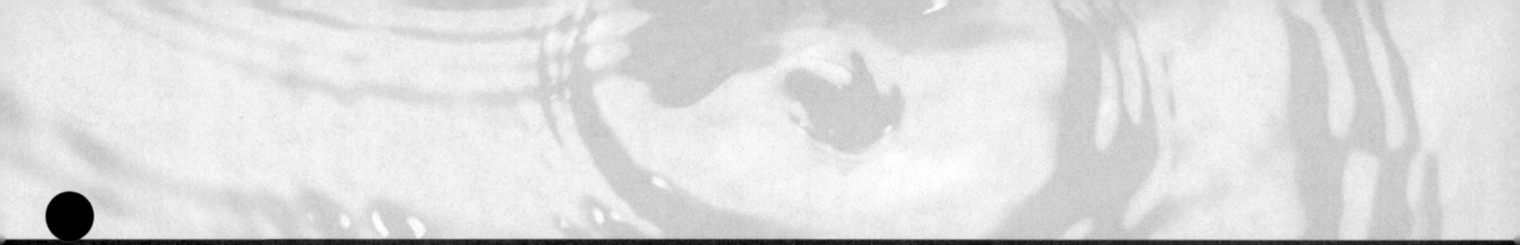

COMMUNITY DISASTER PREPAREDNESS INVENTORY

Description: This inventory is intended to assist the community health nurse and others in the community to assess the community's level of disaster preparedness.

Appropriate populations: This tool can be used to assess disaster preparation in a community or target groups within the community. It can also be adapted to assess disaster preparedness of institutions within the community.

Data sources and data collection strategies: Information used in the assessment may be obtained from local officials or institutional leaders, from a local office of disaster management if one exists, and from interviews with agency personnel and community residents.

Use of information: The information gleaned from the assessment is used by the community health nurse and others to determine the level of community preparedness for response to a disaster event and to direct community disaster planning.

COMMUNITY DISASTER PREPAREDNESS CHECKLIST

	Yes	**No**
Is there a community disaster plan?	❑	❑
If so, is the plan being implemented?	❑	❑
Is there a person in charge of promoting, developing, and coordinating emergency preparation?	❑	❑
Does the disaster plan contain provisions for disaster warning to residents?	❑	❑
Are emergency preparedness activities coordinated among relevant community agencies?	❑	❑
Are all responding agencies and staff familiar with the community disaster plan?	❑	❑
Are community residents familiar with the disaster plan?	❑	❑
Are there operational plans for health response to a disaster?	❑	❑
Have mass casualty plans been developed by local health agencies?	❑	❑
Are surveillance measures in place for early detection and response to health emergencies?	❑	❑
Have steps been taken by environmental health services to prepare for disaster response?	❑	❑
Have facilities and safe areas been designated as shelter sites in the event of a disaster?	❑	❑
Have provisions been made for health care services in shelter sites?	❑	❑
Have health care personnel received disaster preparedness training?	❑	❑
Are resources available for rapid health response to disaster (e.g., communications, financing, transport, supplies)?	❑	❑
Is there a system for updating information on supplies and personnel?	❑	❑
Has the disaster plan been tested?	❑	❑

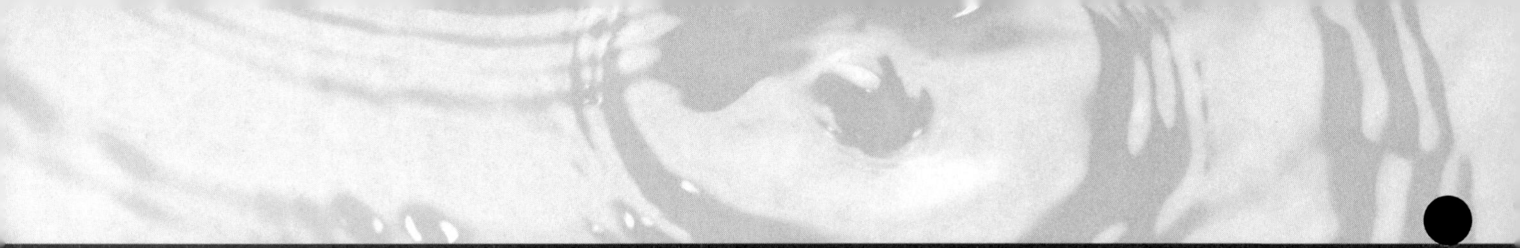

DISASTER ASSESSMENT AND PLANNING GUIDE

Description: This tool is intended to assist community health nurses and other community members to assess the level of disaster preparedness in the community and to plan for effective disaster response. The assessment component of the tool is based on the six dimensions of health in the dimensions model and reflects biophysical, psychological, physical environmental, sociocultural, behavioral, and health system factors influencing disasters and community response to them. Community health nurses and others assessing community disaster preparedness may want to begin the assessment with the *Community Disaster Preparedness Checklist* (p. 121) to identify areas in which more in-depth assessment is required and then use this tool to direct that in-depth assessment.

Appropriate populations: May be used to assess and plan for disaster preparedness at the community level. May also be used to develop disaster plans for specific health care agencies and institutions or other groups within the community (e.g., schools). Some of the questions also address assessment after a disaster event has occurred.

Data sources and data collection strategies: Sources of data for community disaster assessment and planning may include community historical records, official government documents, existing disaster plans of community agencies and organizations, and interviews with key individuals within the community. Additional sources of data may include local businesses and industries, schools, health departments, civil defense/disaster agencies, and the local chapter of the American Red Cross. Information on community resources may also be available from social and civic organizations and clubs. Area maps and personal observation by the community health nurse and others may also provide important information. Because disaster planning should be a community-wide endeavor, community health nurses will be only one group involved in obtaining assessment data and developing a community disaster plan. Community health nurses, however, may create the impetus for disaster planning and/or coordinate data collection and interpretation and disaster response planning.

Use of information: Data obtained using the tool will be used to identify community disaster potential and to plan means of preventing disasters from occurring or mitigating their adverse effects on the community. Assessment data should be used to develop a general plan of community disaster response that would fit many types of disaster events. Assessment data may also serve as an impetus for educating the general public regarding disaster preparedness.

DISASTER ASSESSMENT AND PLANNING GUIDE

Assessment

Biophysical Considerations

What is the age composition of the population(s) most likely to be affected by a disaster? ____________________

Are there special health needs present in the age group(s) identified? ____________________

What is the ethnic/racial composition of the population(s) most likely to be affected by a disaster? What effects, if any, will ethnicity have on response to a disaster? ____________________

What is the extent of injury anticipated as a result of a disaster? What types of injuries are most likely to occur? ____________________

What chronic health problems are prevalent among the population(s) most likely to be affected by a disaster? ____

What communicable disease problems are anticipated as a result of a disaster? ____________________

What currently existing communicable diseases prevalent in the community might complicate disaster response and recovery (e.g., TB, HIV infection)? ____________________

What is the typical rate of pregnancy in the population(s) most likely to be affected by a disaster? ____________

Psychological Considerations

What is the attitude of members of the community toward disaster preparedness? ____________________

How has the community responded to disasters in the past, if any? ____________________

What is the response of community members to disaster warnings? ____________________

What factors are influencing their response? ____________________

What is the extent of the community's ability to cope with the effects of a disaster? ____________________

What is the prevalence of mental illness in the population(s) most likely to be affected by a disaster? ________

What effect is the extent of mental illness likely to have on community disaster response? ____________________

____

What is the extent of loss of life in the disaster? ____________________

What is the extent of deaths subsequent to the disaster? ____________________

____

What is the extent of material loss resulting from the disaster? ____________________

____

What are the psychological effects of the disaster on victims? ____________________

____

What are the psychological effects of the disaster on rescue workers? ____________________

What are the long-term psychological effects of the disaster on the community? ____________________

____

Physical Environmental Considerations

Which of the following physical features of the community create the potential for disaster?

Flooding: ____________________

Forest or brushfires: ____________________

Earthquake: ____________________

Explosion or volcanic eruption: ____________________

Severe weather conditions: ____________________

Other (specify): ____________________

What structures are most/least likely to be damaged in a disaster? ____________________

____

To what extent are vital community structures likely to withstand a disaster? ____________________

____

What community structures could be used as emergency shelters? ____________________

____

What effect are local weather conditions likely to have on community response to a disaster? ____________________

____

Are there elements of the physical environment that might hinder disaster response (blockage of roads)? ________

____

____

Is it likely that a disaster event will threaten community water supplies? ____________________

____

Are animals likely to be involved in a disaster? _______ If so, what effect will this have on human health? ________

____

What is the extent of structural damage resulting from the disaster? ____________________

____

Is there potential for continuing structural damage? _______ Does structural damage pose further risk to victims? _______ To rescuers? _______

Is there a need for shelter for persons displaced by the disaster? _______

Sociocultural Considerations

Do relationships in the community have the potential to create a disaster (e.g., war, civil strife)? _______

How cohesive is the community? _______

Are community members able to work together for disaster planning? _______

Is there potential for conflict between populations most likely to be affected by a disaster? _______

What provisions, if any, have been made for reuniting families separated by a disaster? _______

What social support systems will be available to victims if a disaster occurs? _______

To what extent do community agencies collaborate in disaster planning? _______

What is the extent of knowledge among community residents regarding plans for disaster response? _______

What plans have been made for communicating disaster warnings to residents? _______

Is there a need for special measures to communicate warnings to some groups in the community? _______ If so, what factors contribute to these special needs? _______

Are there language barriers to communicating disaster warnings? _______ If so, what plans have been made to circumvent these barriers? _______

What are the anticipated effects of a disaster on normal channels of communication in the community? _______

What community group/agency is responsible for coordinating disaster planning? _______

How widespread is community participation in disaster planning? _______

To what extent are individual community members/families prepared for disaster events? _______

Who is responsible for activating the community disaster plan? _______

How will the responsible person or group be notified of a disaster? ______

Do community leaders responsible for disaster response activities have high levels of credibility among residents?

______

Do community industries pose disaster hazards? ______ If so, what types of hazards are involved? ______

To what extent do local industries adhere to safety standards? ______

How is adherence monitored? ______

What occupational groups present in the community could assist with disaster response? ______

How will these groups be notified of the need for their assistance? ______

How adequate is the number of rescue personnel available to meet community disaster needs? ______

How adequately have rescue personnel been trained in rescue operations? ______

Is the training of rescue personnel updated periodically? ______

What is the economic status of those affected by disaster? ______

What is the extent of the community's economic capacity for recovery after a disaster? ______

What needs for economic assistance are anticipated following a disaster? ______

How might assistance be obtained? ______

What are the anticipated effects of different types of disasters on the local economy? ______

Is there potential for transportation-related disasters? ______

What is the anticipated effect of the disaster on local transportation? ______

What is the anticipated effect of a disaster on essential community services? ______

What community services are available to assist with disaster recovery? ______

What equipment is available for disaster response? ____________________

Is equipment kept in good working order? ____________________

Have anticipated supplies for effective disaster response been stored at accessible locations throughout the community? _______ Where are supplies stored? ____________________
Are supplies replaced as needed? ____________________

Behavioral Considerations

Do consumption patterns (e.g., smoking, alcohol use) create the potential for disaster? ____________________

What is the extent of substance use and abuse in the community? ____________________
What effect will the extent of substance abuse have on community disaster response? ____________________

What plans have been made to provide food and water for anticipated disaster victims and rescuers? ____________________

How will food and water supplies be dispensed? ____________________

Are there special dietary needs among the population(s) likely to be affected by a disaster? _______ What provisions have been made to meet those needs? ____________________

What community leisure pursuits pose potential disaster hazards? ____________________

Do community members engage in recreational safety measures designed to prevent disasters? ____________________

What leisure pursuits by community members could enhance disaster response capabilities? ____________________

To what extent have psychological effects of the disaster increased the incidence or prevalence of substance abuse in the population? ____________________

Health System Considerations

How well prepared are health service agencies to respond to a disaster? ____________________

What facilities are available to care for disaster victims? ____________________

To what extent is the health system prepared to care for vulnerable populations affected by a disaster (e.g., the elderly, pregnant women, individuals with disabilities)? ____________________

What is the extent of basic first aid and other health-related knowledge in the community? ____________________

What health care personnel are available to meet health needs in a disaster (*consider both emergency and routine service needs*)? ____________________

How will they be mobilized to respond? ____________________

What is the anticipated effect of a disaster on health care services? ____________________

What steps have been taken to minimize disruption of services? ____________________

What health care needs are anticipated as a result of a disaster? ____________________

What plans have been made to meet those needs? ____________________

What plans have been made to support triage activities? ____________________

What plans have been made for creating medical treatment areas? ____________________

What plans have been made for transporting victims to treatment areas? ____________________

What medications are likely to be needed by victims of a disaster? ____________________

Have supplies of essential medications been stored in accessible locations? ____________________

What medical and first aid supplies will be needed for disaster response? ____________________

What supplies will be needed for health care in shelters? ____________________

Have supplies been obtained and stored in accessible locations? ____________________

How will medications and supplies be transported to areas of need? ____________________

How will medications and supplies be dispensed? ____________________

Have plans been made for the identification of the dead? _______ For notifying family members? _______ For disposing of bodies? _______ What do these plans entail? ____________________

What mental health services will be available immediately following a disaster and during the recovery period?

____

Diagnosis and Planning

Community Disaster Potential

Type of Potential Disaster	Contributing Factors

Vulnerable Populations

Population	Source of Vulnerability

Disaster Prevention/Mitigation Activities

Disaster Prevention Activities	Disaster Mitigation Activities

Anticipated Disaster-Related Health Problems and Planned Interventions

Anticipated Problem	Planned Intervention

Disaster Plan Elements

Mechanisms for warning residents: ____________________

Mechanisms for initiating disaster plan implementation: ____________________

Plans for communication: ____________________

Procedures for traffic control and transportation of equipment, supplies, and personnel to the disaster site: ____________________

Procedures for evacuating residents: ____________________

Plans for rescue operations: ____________________

Plans for damage inventory: ____________________

Plans for mobilizing health care providers: ____________________

Plans for injury assessment: ____________________

Plans for meeting immediate care needs of disaster victims: ____________________

Plans for providing shelter: ____________________

Plans for shelter governance: ______

Plans for providing supportive care: ______

Plans for public health surveillance: ______

Mechanisms to assist victims during the recovery period: ______

Mechanisms for evaluating the adequacy of the disaster plan: ______

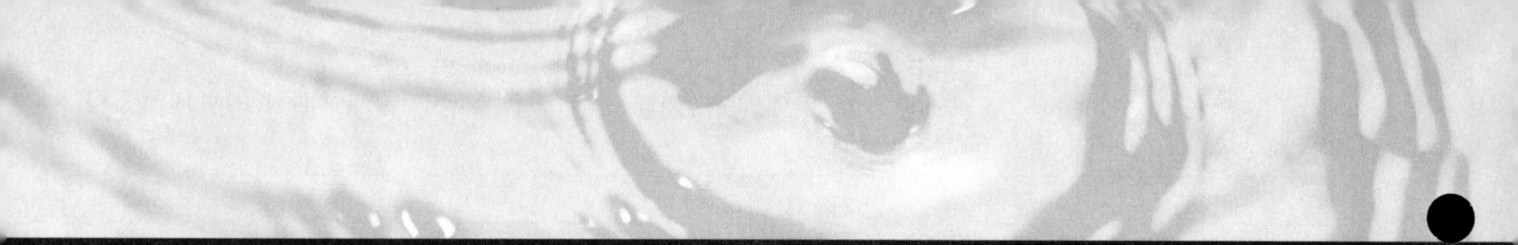

COMMUNICABLE DISEASE RISK FACTOR INVENTORY

Description: This inventory is intended to assist the community health nurse to identify individual clients or population groups at risk for communicable diseases. Risk factors in each of the six dimensions of health are addressed.

Appropriate populations: May be used with individual clients or population groups to identify risk factors for communicable diseases amenable to modification. Appropriate to all age groups and ethnic/cultural groups.

Data sources and data collection strategies: For individual clients, most of the information addressed in the inventory will be obtained from interviews with the client or significant others. Some information may also be available in existing health records (e.g., history of treatment for sexually transmitted disease). Information related to population groups will come from a variety of sources including local health department statistics, records of local health care providers, school records, and data on absenteeism from local industries and businesses. Additional information may be obtained in interviews with or surveys of community residents or major informants such as health care providers, community officials, and so on.

Use of information: Risk factors identified in the use of the inventory provide a starting point for client education and efforts to modify risk factors to prevent the occurrence of communicable diseases or to limit their effects on individuals or population groups. Based on his or her knowledge of the contribution of specific types of risk factors to certain communicable diseases, the community health nurse explores with the client the risk of communicable disease and ways to modify risk factors to prevent disease or mitigate its effects. For example, if the client has multiple sexual partners and engages in injection drug use, the community health nurse would determine that he or she is at high risk for HIV infection; hepatitis B, C, and D; and sexually transmitted diseases. The nurse would then educate the client regarding the increased risk for these diseases and suggest ways of eliminating or modifying risk factors. Information on risk factors in the population would be used to plan programs designed to eliminate or modify the identified risks for communicable diseases.

COMMUNICABLE DISEASE RISK FACTOR INVENTORY

Item *(Note: The "client" may be an individual or a group of people.)*	**Yes**	**No**
Biophysical Considerations		
Is the client (population) in an age group at particular risk for:		
Measles?	❑	❑
Mumps?	❑	❑
Rubella?	❑	❑
Diphtheria?	❑	❑
Pertussis?	❑	❑
Tetanus?	❑	❑
Poliomyelitis?	❑	❑
HiB disease?	❑	❑
Hepatitis A?	❑	❑
Hepatitis B?	❑	❑
HIV infection?	❑	❑
Sexually transmitted diseases?	❑	❑
Tuberculosis?	❑	❑
Influenza?	❑	❑
Varicella?	❑	❑
Does the client have an existing chronic disease?	❑	❑
Is the client receiving immunosuppressive therapy?	❑	❑
Does the client have HIV infection?	❑	❑
Is the client overly fatigued?	❑	❑
Is the client pregnant?	❑	❑
Does the client have a history of sexually transmitted diseases?	❑	❑
Has the client received blood or blood products?	❑	❑
Does the client have symptoms suggestive of disease?	❑	❑
Psychological Considerations		
Is the client under stress?	❑	❑
Is the client depressed?	❑	❑
Does the client have a poor self-image that would lead to high-risk behaviors?	❑	❑
Is there a history of past trauma that might lead to increased risk of disease?	❑	❑
Does the presence of mental illness increase the risk of disease?	❑	❑
Does the disease have potential psychological consequences?	❑	❑
Physical Environmental Considerations		
Does the client live in crowded conditions?	❑	❑
Is the client at risk for insect or animal bite?	❑	❑
Do elements of the physical environment serve as sources of exposure to communicable disease?	❑	❑
Do physical environmental conditions contribute to the presence of animal or insect disease vectors?	❑	❑
Is the client exposed to contaminated food or water?	❑	❑
Is the client exposed to poor sanitary conditions?	❑	❑
Do seasonal variations affect the risk of disease?	❑	❑
Do environmental factors impede access to diagnostic or treatment services?	❑	❑
Sociocultural Considerations		
Is the client homeless?	❑	❑
Does the client live in a shelter or other institutional setting?	❑	❑
Is the client subjected to peer pressure for high-risk behaviors?	❑	❑

Item (*Note: The "client" may be an individual or a group of people.*)	**Yes**	**No**
Do social mores support high-risk behaviors?	❑	❑
Are family members or friends ill?	❑	❑
Does the client's occupation increase the risk of disease?	❑	❑
If in a high-risk occupation, does the client use universal precautions?	❑	❑
Is the client involved in childcare (*as recipient or provider*)?	❑	❑
Do cultural beliefs and behaviors increase the client's risk of disease?	❑	❑
Does the client live in an area where communicable disease is endemic?	❑	❑
Does the client travel to areas where communicable disease is endemic?	❑	❑
Do societal attitudes to the disease hamper control efforts?	❑	❑
Is there social stigma attached to the disease that may hamper control efforts?	❑	❑
Do media messages affect risk behaviors for or attitudes toward the disease?	❑	❑
Does socioeconomic status influence risk of the disease?	❑	❑
Does education level influence risk of disease?	❑	❑
Does gender socialization affect disease risk?	❑	❑
Does the disease have potential as a bioterrorist threat?	❑	❑
Behavioral Considerations		
Is the client malnourished?	❑	❑
Does the client engage in substance abuse?	❑	❑
Does the client use injectable drugs?	❑	❑
Does the client share drug paraphernalia?	❑	❑
Does the client frequent "shooting galleries"?	❑	❑
Is the client sexually active?	❑	❑
Does the client have multiple sexual partners?	❑	❑
Does the client use safe sexual practices?	❑	❑
Does the client engage in regular condom use with sexual activity?	❑	❑
Does the client douche?	❑	❑
Does the client use oral contraceptives?	❑	❑
Does the client engage in prostitution for drugs or money?	❑	❑
Does the client have sexual intercourse with members of high-risk groups?	❑	❑
Does the client use good personal hygiene practices (e.g., handwashing)?	❑	❑
Does the client wash fruits and vegetables thoroughly before eating them?	❑	❑
Does the client cook foods sufficiently to kill any microorganisms?	❑	❑
Does the client purify contaminated water before drinking or cooking?	❑	❑
Health System Considerations		
Is the client adequately immunized against:		
Measles?	❑	❑
Mumps?	❑	❑
Rubella?	❑	❑
Diphtheria?	❑	❑
Pertussis?	❑	❑
Tetanus?	❑	❑
HiB disease?	❑	❑
Hepatitis A?	❑	❑
Hepatitis B?	❑	❑
Human papillomavirus (HPV)?	❑	❑
Varicella?	❑	❑
Influenza?	❑	❑
Tuberculosis?	❑	❑
Can the client afford immunization services?	❑	❑
Does the client's insurance cover immunization services?	❑	❑
Are health care providers conversant with the signs and symptoms of disease?	❑	❑

Item (*Note: The "client" may be an individual or a group of people.*)	**Yes**	**No**
Do health provider behaviors contribute to disease (e.g., overuse of antibiotics)?	❑	❑
Do routine medical interventions contribute to disease risk?	❑	❑
Are diagnostic and treatment services readily available?	❑	❑
Do provider attitudes to persons with the disease affect willingness to seek treatment?	❑	❑

CHRONIC DISEASE RISK FACTOR INVENTORY

Description: This inventory is intended to assist the community health nurse to identify individual clients or population groups at risk for common chronic conditions. Risk factors in each of the six dimensions of health are addressed.

Appropriate populations: May be used with individual clients or population groups to identify risk factors amenable to modification. Appropriate to all age groups and cultural groups.

Data sources and data collection strategies: For individual clients, most of the information addressed in the inventory will be obtained from interviews with the client or significant others. Some information may also be available in existing health records. Information related to population groups will come from a variety of sources including local health department statistics, records of local health care providers, school records, and data on absenteeism from local industries and businesses. Additional information may be obtained in interviews with or surveys of community residents or major informants such as health care providers, community officials, and so on.

Use of information: Risk factors identified in the use of the inventory provide a starting point for client education and efforts to modify risk factors to prevent the occurrence of chronic conditions or to limit their effects on individuals or population groups. Based on his or her knowledge of the contribution of specific types of risk factors to certain chronic conditions, the community health nurse explores with the client the risk of disease and ways to modify risk factors to prevent disease or mitigate its effects. For example, if the client has a family history of lung cancer and smokes, the community health nurse would determine that this individual is at high risk for lung cancer and other chronic conditions such as heart disease. The nurse would then educate the client regarding the increased risk of these diseases and suggest ways of eliminating or modifying risk factors. Similar kinds of actions might be taken to modify population risk factors.

CHRONIC DISEASE RISK FACTOR INVENTORY

Item (*Note: The "client" may be an individual or a group of people.*)	Yes	No
Biophysical Considerations		
Is the client (population) in an age group at particular risk for chronic health problems?	❑	❑
Does the client have a family history of hereditary chronic health problems?	❑	❑
Does the client have an existing condition that increases the risk of other chronic problems?	❑	❑
Does the client have physical problems that increase the risk of accidental injury?	❑	❑
Is the client overweight?	❑	❑
Does the client have hypertension?	❑	❑
Does the client have asthma or RAD?	❑	❑
Does the condition have the potential for functional limitations?	❑	❑
Has the client been immunized against HPV?	❑	❑
Psychological Considerations		
Is the client under stress?	❑	❑
Do existing psychological problems impede control of the chronic disease?	❑	❑
Has adaptation to the chronic disease occurred?	❑	❑
Physical Environmental Considerations		
Is the client exposed to environmental pollutants?	❑	❑
Do environmental conditions increase the risk of accidental injury?	❑	❑
Is the client exposed to high noise levels?	❑	❑
Is the client exposed to temperature extremes?	❑	❑
Is the client exposed to high levels of ionizing radiation?	❑	❑
Does the condition require modification of the physical environment?	❑	❑
Sociocultural Considerations		
Do societal norms support behaviors that increase the risk of chronic health problems?	❑	❑
Do the client's peers support behaviors that increase the risk of chronic health problems?	❑	❑
Do economic or educational factors affect risk for the condition?	❑	❑
Is there social stigma attached to the condition?	❑	❑
Do social attitudes to the chronic condition impede control?	❑	❑
Do cultural beliefs and behaviors increase the risk of chronic health problems?	❑	❑
Does legislation affect the risk of chronic health problems?	❑	❑
Does the client's occupation increase the risk of disease?	❑	❑
If in a high-risk occupation, does the client engage in preventive measures at work?	❑	❑
Behavioral Considerations		
Does the client's diet increase the risk of chronic health problems?	❑	❑
Does the chronic condition necessitate dietary changes?	❑	❑
Does the client smoke or use other forms of tobacco?	❑	❑
Does the client use drugs or alcohol that increase the risk of chronic health problems?	❑	❑
Does the client have a sedentary lifestyle?	❑	❑
Do self-care practices (e.g., mammogram) decrease the risk of death from chronic health problems?	❑	❑
Do sexual practices increase the risk of chronic health problems (e.g., multiple sexual partners increases risk of cervical cancer)?	❑	❑
Does the client use sunscreen or wear protective clothing outdoors?	❑	❑
Does the client use safety equipment (e.g., seat belts, hearing protection)?	❑	❑
Does the client engage in recreational activities that increase the risk for chronic health problems?	❑	❑
Does the chronic condition necessitate regular medication use?	❑	❑
Does the chronic condition necessitate other self-care behaviors (e.g., glucose monitoring)?	❑	❑

Item *(Note: The "client" may be an individual or a group of people.)*	**Yes**	**No**
Health System Considerations		
Does the client receive routine screening for chronic health problems?	❑	❑
Has the client been educated regarding risk factors for chronic health problems?	❑	❑
Does the client comply with treatment recommendations for conditions that increase the risk of chronic health problems?	❑	❑
Does the client take medications that increase the risk of accidental injury?	❑	❑
Do health system factors contribute to increased risk of disease?	❑	❑
Are screening, diagnostic, and treatment services available for the condition?	❑	❑
Are alternative therapies available and used for the condition?	❑	❑
Do attitudes of providers to persons with the condition impede control efforts?	❑	❑

MENTAL ILLNESS RISK FACTOR INVENTORY

Description: This inventory is intended to assist the community health nurse to identify clients or population groups at risk for or exhibiting symptoms of mental illness. Influencing factors in the biophysical, psychological, physical environmental, sociocultural, behavioral, and health systems dimensions of health are addressed.

Appropriate populations: May be used with individual clients or population groups to identify risk factors amenable to modification. Appropriate to all age groups and cultural groups.

Data sources and data collection strategies: For individual clients, most of the information addressed in the inventory will be obtained from interviews with the client or significant others. Some information may also be available in existing health records. Information related to population groups will come from a variety of sources including local mental health agencies and local health care providers. Additional information may be obtained in interviews with or surveys of community residents or major informants such as health care providers, community officials, and so on.

Use of information: Risk factors identified using the inventory can guide client education and risk factor modification to prevent the occurrence of mental illness. Risk factor information may also be used to design community programs to prevent or treat mental illness.

MENTAL ILLNESS RISK FACTOR INVENTORY

Item *(Note: The "client" may be an individual or a group of people.)*	**Yes**	**No**
Biophysical Considerations		
Is there a family history of mental health problems?	❑	❑
Is the client experiencing physical health problems that may contribute to mental health problems?	❑	❑
Do family members have physical health problems that may lead to caregiver burden and mental health problems?	❑	❑
Do physical health problems or their treatment cause signs and symptoms suggestive of mental health problems?	❑	❑
Does the presence of a mental health problem complicate treatment of physical health conditions?	❑	❑
Psychological Considerations		
Is the client experiencing high levels of stress?	❑	❑
Does stress contribute to or exacerbate existing mental health problems?	❑	❑
Does the client exhibit effective coping strategies?	❑	❑
Does the client exhibit signs and symptoms that suggest the presence of mental health problems?	❑	❑
Has the client adapted to the presence of an existing mental health problem?	❑	❑
Is there existing psychiatric comorbidity?	❑	❑
Is the client at risk for suicide as a result of the mental health problem?	❑	❑
Physical Environmental Considerations		
Does the client exhibit seasonal mood changes?	❑	❑
Has the client been exposed to pollutants that may contribute to mental health problems?	❑	❑
Sociocultural Considerations		
Have mental health problems affected the client's social interactions (with family or others)?	❑	❑
Has the client experienced social stigma due to mental health problems?	❑	❑
Do the client's cultural beliefs affect perceptions of mental health problems or willingness to seek help?	❑	❑
Do mental health problems contribute to the risk of homelessness for the client?	❑	❑
Does the client have an adequate social support system?	❑	❑
Is the client employed?	❑	❑
Does job stress increase the risk of mental health problems?	❑	❑
Does mental illness affect the client's ability to work?	❑	❑
Behavioral Considerations		
Does the client use alcohol, drugs, or tobacco in an effort to self-manage symptoms?	❑	❑
Does exercise assist with control of the mental health problem?	❑	❑
Does tobacco use influence the problem?	❑	❑
Does the problem affect self-care behaviors?	❑	❑
Health System Considerations		
Does the client have access to treatment for mental health problems?	❑	❑
Does the client have health insurance coverage for mental health services?	❑	❑
Are health care providers alert to signs and symptoms of mental health problems?	❑	❑
Does the client comply with treatment recommendations?	❑	❑

Item *(Note: The "client" may be an individual or a group of people.)*	**Yes**	**No**
Does the client exhibit treatment side effects or adverse effects?	❑	❑
Does treatment for other health problems cause or exacerbate the mental health problem?	❑	❑
Do health care provider attitudes to mental illness impede control?	❑	❑

SUBSTANCE ABUSE RISK FACTOR INVENTORY

Description: This inventory is intended to assist the community health nurse to identify clients or population groups at risk for substance abuse. Risk factors in the biophysical, psychological, sociocultural, behavioral, and health systems dimensions of health are addressed.

Appropriate populations: May be used with individual clients or population groups to identify risk factors amenable to modification. Appropriate to all age groups and cultural groups.

Data sources and data collection strategies: For individual clients, most of the information addressed in the inventory will be obtained from interviews with the client or significant others. Some information may also be available in existing health records. Information related to population groups will come from a variety of sources including local police and insurance statistics and records of local health care providers. Additional information may be obtained in interviews with or surveys of community residents or major informants such as health care providers, community officials, and so on.

Use of information: Risk factors identified in the use of the inventory provide a starting point for client education and efforts to modify risk factors to prevent the occurrence of substance abuse. Risk factor information may also be used to design community programs to prevent substance abuse.

SUBSTANCE ABUSE RISK FACTOR INVENTORY

Item (*Note: The "client" may be an individual or a group of people.*)	**Yes**	**No**
Biophysical Considerations		
Is the client (population) in an age group at particular risk for substance abuse?	☐	☐
Does the client have a family history of substance abuse?	☐	☐
Does the client have an existing physical condition that might lead to substance abuse?	☐	☐
Does the client exhibit periodic signs of intoxication?	☐	☐
Does the client exhibit periodic signs of withdrawal?	☐	☐
Does the client exhibit signs and symptoms of long-term effects of substance abuse?	☐	☐
Is the client pregnant?	☐	☐
Does the client have a history of fetal exposure to psychoactive substances?	☐	☐
Does the client have difficulty sleeping?	☐	☐
Psychological Considerations		
Is the client under stress?	☐	☐
Does the client have a poor self-image?	☐	☐
Does the client have realistic life goals?	☐	☐
Does the client exhibit poor impulse control?	☐	☐
Does the client have poor coping skills?	☐	☐
Is the client depressed?	☐	☐
Has the client experienced a recent significant loss?	☐	☐
Does the client have a history of mental or emotional illness?	☐	☐
Does the client currently exhibit signs of other psychopathology?	☐	☐
Sociocultural Considerations		
Do community norms support substance abuse?	☐	☐
Do the client's peers support substance abuse?	☐	☐
Is alcohol or drug use a regular part of social interaction?	☐	☐
Are drugs and alcohol easily accessible?	☐	☐
Is legislation regarding drug and alcohol access enforced?	☐	☐
Do cultural or religious values influence drug or alcohol use?	☐	☐
Is the client unemployed?	☐	☐
Is the client experiencing financial difficulties?	☐	☐
Is the client subjected to discrimination?	☐	☐
Do occupational factors increase the client's risk of substance abuse?	☐	☐
Does the client have a history of frequent work or school absence?	☐	☐
Has the client had difficulty meeting work or school expectations?	☐	☐
Is the client experiencing difficulty in interpersonal interactions?	☐	☐
Is the client experiencing difficulty in family interactions?	☐	☐
Do family members exhibit co-dependence?	☐	☐
Has the client been a victim or perpetrator of family violence?	☐	☐
Does the client engage in violent behavior?	☐	☐
Is the client socially isolated?	☐	☐
Is the client homeless?	☐	☐
Is the client engaged in criminal activity related to drugs or alcohol?	☐	☐
Behavioral Considerations		
Does the client report a loss of appetite?	☐	☐
Does the client smoke or use other forms of tobacco?	☐	☐
Does the client use drugs recreationally?	☐	☐
Is drug or alcohol use associated with leisure activities?	☐	☐
Does the client engage in other high-risk behaviors (e.g., driving while intoxicated)?	☐	☐
Does the client engage in prostitution for drugs?	☐	☐

Item (*Note: The "client" may be an individual or a group of people.*)	**Yes**	**No**
Health System Considerations		
Has the client received prescriptions for psychoactive drugs?	❑	❑
Does the client have a history of past substance abuse treatment?	❑	❑
Do providers assess for signs of substance abuse?	❑	❑
Do providers engage in brief interventions for clients at risk for substance abuse?	❑	❑
Does the client have access to treatment for substance abuse?	❑	❑
Is there adequate funding for treatment for substance abuse?	❑	❑

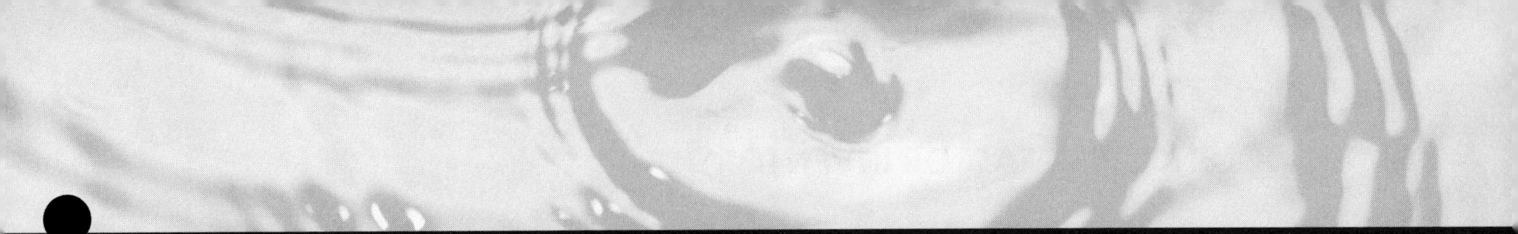

FAMILY VIOLENCE RISK FACTOR INVENTORY

Description: This inventory is intended to assist the community health nurse to identify clients or population groups at risk for family violence. The inventory assesses risk for all forms of family violence, including child abuse, intimate partner violence, and elder abuse. Risk factors in the biophysical, psychological, sociocultural, behavioral, and health system dimensions of health are addressed.

Appropriate populations: May be used with individual clients or population groups to identify risk factors amenable to modification. Appropriate to all age groups and cultural groups.

Data sources and data collection strategies: For individual clients, most of the information addressed in the inventory will be obtained from interviews with the client or significant others. Some information may also be available in existing health or protective services records. Information related to population groups will come from a variety of sources including local police and health agency records and news media. Additional information may be obtained in interviews with or surveys of community residents or major informants such as health care providers, community officials, and so on.

Use of information: Risk factors identified in the use of the inventory provide a starting point for client and community education and efforts to modify risk factors to prevent the occurrence of family violence. Risk factor information may also be used to design community programs to prevent violence.

FAMILY VIOLENCE RISK FACTOR INVENTORY

Item (*Note: The "client" may be a specific family or a population group.)*	**Yes**	**No**
Biophysical Considerations		
Are family members in age groups at particular risk for abuse?	❑	❑
Do family members have existing physical conditions that increase the risk of violence?	❑	❑
Is there physical evidence of neglect or abuse in family members?	❑	❑
Is a member of the family pregnant?	❑	❑
Is there a history of head trauma in a family member?	❑	❑
Psychological Considerations		
Are family members under stress?	❑	❑
Do family members have poor self-concepts?	❑	❑
Do family members have poor coping skills?	❑	❑
Do family members exhibit poor impulse control?	❑	❑
Are family members depressed?	❑	❑
Is there a negative emotional climate in the family?	❑	❑
Is there a family history of mental or emotional illness?	❑	❑
Do family members exhibit annoying traits?	❑	❑
Are expectations of family members unrealistic?	❑	❑
Do some family members have excessive power over others?	❑	❑
Sociocultural Considerations		
Do community norms support family violence?	❑	❑
Do significant others support family violence?	❑	❑
Have family members been subject to past abuse?	❑	❑
Are family interactions positive?	❑	❑
Is the family experiencing financial difficulty?	❑	❑
Do cultural or religious values influence the risk of violence?	❑	❑
Are one or more family members unemployed?	❑	❑
Is the family socially isolated?	❑	❑
Does the family have an inadequate social support network?	❑	❑
Is there evidence of emotional or economic dependence among family members?	❑	❑
Is there an occupational risk for violence victimization?	❑	❑
Is there a perception of social stigma attached to being a victim of violence?	❑	❑
Is there social unrest in the population that may contribute to increased violence?	❑	❑
Behavioral Considerations		
Do family members use or abuse alcohol?	❑	❑
Do family members use or abuse drugs?	❑	❑
Is one family member excessively sexually dominant?	❑	❑
Is cohabitation present in the family?	❑	❑
Does sexual orientation or gender identity contribute to the potential for violence?	❑	❑
Do other behaviors contribute to risk of violence (e.g., fighting)?	❑	❑
Health System Considerations		
Do family members make frequent use of health services (especially emergency services)?	❑	❑
Do family members have a regular source of health care?	❑	❑
Do health or medical care needs create stress for family members?	❑	❑
Do health care providers assess for violence?	❑	❑
Are support services available for victims and perpetrators of violence?	❑	❑

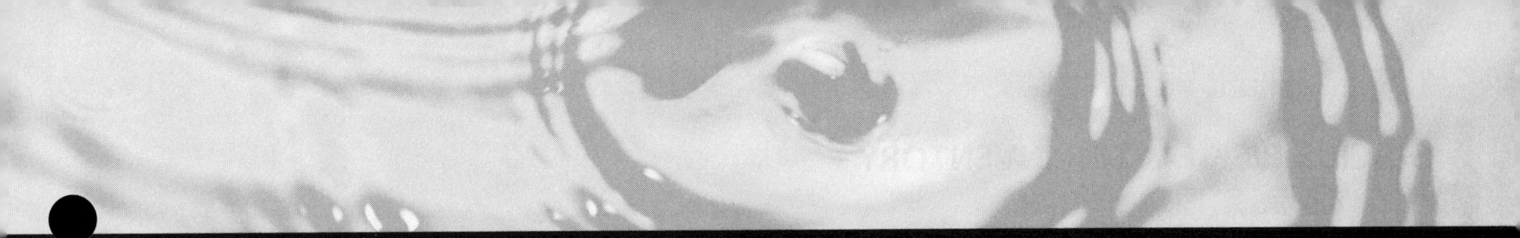

SUICIDE RISK FACTOR INVENTORY

Description: This inventory is intended to assist the community health nurse to identify clients or population groups at risk for suicide. Risk factors in each of the six dimensions of health are addressed.

Appropriate populations: May be used with individual clients or population groups to identify risk factors amenable to modification. Appropriate to all age groups and cultural groups.

Data sources and data collection strategies: For individual clients, most of the information addressed in the inventory will be obtained from interviews with the client or significant others. Some information may also be available in existing health records. Information related to population groups will come from a variety of sources including local police and insurance statistics and records of local health care providers. Additional information may be obtained in interviews with or surveys of community residents or major informants such as health care providers, community officials, and so on.

Use of information: Risk factors identified in the use of the inventory enable the community health nurse to initiate interventions to prevent suicide by individual clients. Risk factor information may also be used to design community programs to prevent suicide.

SUICIDE RISK FACTOR INVENTORY

Item (*Note: The "client" may be an individual or a group of people.)*	**Yes**	**No**
Biophysical Considerations		
Is the client (population) in an age group at particular risk for suicide?	❑	❑
Does the client have an existing physical condition that might lead to suicide?	❑	❑
Is the client experiencing a developmental or maturational crisis (e.g., adolescence)?	❑	❑
Is the client experiencing significant pain?	❑	❑
Does the client report insomnia?	❑	❑
Psychological Considerations		
Is the client under stress?	❑	❑
Does the client have poor coping skills?	❑	❑
Does the client have a poor self-concept?	❑	❑
Does the client have unrealistic expectations of self?	❑	❑
Has the client recently experienced what he or she perceives as a failure?	❑	❑
Is the client depressed?	❑	❑
Has the client experienced a recent significant loss?	❑	❑
Does the client have a history of mental or emotional illness?	❑	❑
Has the client expressed feelings of hopelessness or despair?	❑	❑
Does the client exhibit evidence of anxiety, irritability, or panic?	❑	❑
Does the client fail to refer to future goals or activities?	❑	❑
Has the client made efforts to "put his or her house in order"?	❑	❑
Has the client expressed suicidal thoughts or intentions?	❑	❑
Does the client describe specific plans for suicide?	❑	❑
Has the client made a previous suicide attempt?	❑	❑
Physical Environmental Considerations		
Does the client experience seasonal affective disorder?	❑	❑
Sociocultural Considerations		
Has a friend or family member attempted or completed suicide?	❑	❑
Has the client been exposed to suicide or a suicide attempt by others (*personally or via media coverage*)?	❑	❑
Has the client been a victim of abuse?	❑	❑
Is the client experiencing family or interpersonal difficulties?	❑	❑
Has the client exhibited poor work or school performance?	❑	❑
Does the client have easy access to lethal methods of suicide?	❑	❑
Does the client engage in behaviors designed to result in death (e.g., provoking fights)?	❑	❑
Is the client unemployed?	❑	❑
Is the client experiencing financial difficulties?	❑	❑
Is the client socially isolated?	❑	❑
Is the client homeless?	❑	❑
Behavioral Considerations		
Does the client report a loss of appetite?	❑	❑
Does the client abuse alcohol or drugs?	❑	❑
Does the client engage in regular exercise?	❑	❑
Does the client have any leisure activities?	❑	❑
Health System Considerations		
Does the client have a regular source of health care?	❑	❑
Are health care providers alert to signs of impending suicide?	❑	❑
Are suicide prevention services available in the community?	❑	❑